CertiPrep – BACB-RBT Exam Prep Book 2025–2026

CertiPrep

Published by CertiPrep Publishing, 2025.

CERTIPREP – BACB-RBT EXAM PREP BOOK 2025–2026

First edition. November 10, 2025.

ISBN: 979-8232755720

Written by CertiPrep.

Table of Contents

Disclaimer

This book is an independent study resource to help candidates prepare for the Registered Behavior Technician® (RBT®) certification exam. It is not sponsored, endorsed, or approved by the Behavior Analyst Certification Board® (BACB®). The BACB may update RBT eligibility criteria, the RBT Task List, the RBT Ethics Code, and exam policies at any time. You are responsible for checking the most current RBT Handbook, RBT Task List (2nd ed.), and RBT Ethics Code (2.0) on the BACB website before you sit for the exam.

Every reasonable effort has been made to ensure the accuracy and usefulness of the information in this book at the time of writing, but the authors and publisher cannot guarantee that all information will remain current or error-free. Using this book does not guarantee a passing score. Your results will depend on your training, supervision quality, practical experience, and study habits. "Registered Behavior Technician®," "RBT®," "BACB®," and related marks are registered trademarks of the Behavior Analyst Certification Board. This book is independent of the BACB and is not sponsored, endorsed, or affiliated with the Board.

Introduction to the CertiPrep – BACB-RBT Exam Prep Book 2025–2026

The Registered Behavior Technician® (RBT®) is a **paraprofessional-level** credential in applied behavior analysis (ABA). RBTs work directly with clients, implementing behavior-analytic services under the close, ongoing supervision of BCBAs, BCaBAs, or other qualified supervisors. If your daily work includes following behavior plans, taking data, running teaching programs, and supporting clients in clinics, homes, schools, or community settings, this credential is designed for you.

This book is written to match your other CertiPrep exam books: friendly, practical, and focused on how the exam actually tests you. Instead of listing terms alphabetically, each chapter follows the RBT Task List content areas and explains what safe, ethical, entry-level performance looks like in real sessions. You will see concise explanations, short lists that highlight key ideas, and practice questions that feel similar in style to actual exam items.

As of this edition, the RBT exam is based on the **RBT Task List (2nd ed.)** and includes 85 multiple-choice questions (75 scored, 10 unscored pilot items) with a 90-minute time limit. The questions align with six core content areas: Measurement, Assessment, Skill Acquisition, Behavior Reduction, Documentation and Reporting, and Professional Conduct and Scope of Practice. You must also complete the 40-hour RBT training, pass a Competency Assessment, and meet BACB background and supervision requirements before certification.

Who This Book Is For

THIS BOOK IS DESIGNED for people who are actively moving toward the RBT credential or who want a structured, exam-focused overview of the RBT role. If you work as a behavior technician, therapist, paraprofessional, classroom aide, or direct-care staff in ABA organizations, you are exactly the intended audience. You do not need a degree in psychology or behavior analysis to benefit from this book, but you should be comfortable with basic reading, following procedures, and multiple-choice testing.

You will get the most out of this book if you are also enrolled in an approved 40-hour RBT training and working with a qualified supervisor. The chapters are meant to reinforce and organize what you are already seeing in training and in sessions. Even if you are a career changer or new hire with limited experience, the explanations start at a practical, beginner level and build up gradually toward exam-style thinking.

How This Book Is Organized

THE STRUCTURE OF THIS book mirrors your other CertiPrep titles so the layout feels familiar and easy to scan. Content is grouped into parts that match the RBT Task List content areas, with each chapter focusing on a set of closely related skills or responsibilities. Within each chapter, you will see numbered sections (for example, 1.1–1.10) that break concepts into small chunks you can study in short sessions.

Each core chapter includes a short introduction, ten structured sections, and a set of practice questions with an answer key and brief justifications. The language is plain, and explanations are tied to what technicians actually do: taking data, following plans, and communicating with supervisors and caregivers. Later in the book, you will find two full-length mock exams (A and B) so you can test your readiness under exam-like conditions.

How to Use This Book

THE MOST EFFECTIVE way to use this book is as a **structured study guide**, not as something you skim right before test day. For each chapter, read through the sections from start to finish, paying special attention to definitions, ethics points, and "what should the RBT do next" patterns. Then, answer the practice questions at the end of the chapter without looking at the answer key.

When you check your answers, mark any questions you missed or guessed on, and note which topics felt fuzzy. Go back to the relevant sections, re-read them, and write short notes or flashcards in your own words. After you have completed all the content chapters, take one of two full mock exams in one sitting with a 90-minute timer and no notes. Use your results to identify weaker domains and return to those chapters for targeted review.

Exam-Day Tips for RBT Candidates

ON EXAM DAY, LOGISTICS matter just as much as content. Make sure you know whether you are testing at a Pearson VUE center or via online proctoring, what identification you need, and how early you should arrive or log in. Review the current RBT Handbook so you understand check-in, security procedures, and what you can and cannot bring with you.

During the exam, you will have roughly a minute per question, so avoid getting stuck on a single item. Read each question carefully, watching for words like "BEST," "FIRST," "MOST ethical," or "WITHIN the RBT's scope." Eliminate options that ask you to act outside your role, ignore the behavior plan, change treatment without supervision, or violate the RBT Ethics Code. In many questions, the safest choice involves collecting accurate data, following written plans, protecting client dignity, and contacting your supervisor when something serious or unexpected occurs.

Chapter 1: RBT Exam Overview and ABA Fundamentals

The first chapter gives you a foundation for everything else in the book. You will see how the RBT exam is structured, what ABA means in practice, and how the RBT fits into the clinical team. You will also meet core terms such as behavior, antecedent, consequence, reinforcement, and the common functions of behavior that show up in almost every domain of the exam.

If you understand this chapter well, later topics like measurement, skill acquisition, and behavior reduction will feel like a natural extension rather than a set of disconnected rules. Many exam items in other sections quietly depend on these fundamentals, especially questions about ethics, scope of practice, and interpreting simple behavior scenarios.

1.1 The RBT Certification and Exam Snapshot

THE RBT CERTIFICATION is designed as an **entry-level credential** in behavior analysis for people who implement ABA services directly with clients. You work under close, ongoing supervision and do not design treatment plans yourself. The exam checks whether you can perform essential tasks safely, ethically, and consistently according to the RBT Task List.

Key ideas about the RBT exam:

- Paraprofessional certification focused on direct service
- Based on the RBT Task List (2nd ed.) and Ethics Code
- Computer-based exam with fixed length and timing

The RBT is a paraprofessional role, which means you are not expected to make high-level clinical decisions but you are expected to implement plans accurately in real-world settings. The exam blueprint is driven by the RBT Task List (2nd ed.), covering measurement, assessment, skill acquisition, behavior reduction, documentation and reporting, and professional conduct and scope of practice. Ethics expectations are embedded throughout, so questions often test both technical skills and ethical judgment at the same time. The exam is delivered via computer-based testing, includes 85 multiple-choice items, and must be completed in 90 minutes, so pacing and careful reading are essential for success.

1.2 What Is Applied Behavior Analysis (ABA)?

APPLIED BEHAVIOR ANALYSIS (ABA) is a science focused on understanding and improving behavior that matters in everyday life. Instead of guessing about internal states, ABA emphasizes observable behavior and the environmental events that influence it. As an RBT, you are part of the team that uses these principles to help clients build skills and reduce harmful or interfering behaviors.

Core ABA characteristics:

- Focus on observable, measurable behavior
- Emphasis on relationships between environment and behavior
- Data-based decision-making about interventions

Focusing on observable behavior means you pay attention to actions you can see and measure, such as "raises hand," "hits," or "completes worksheet," rather than labels like "lazy" or "stubborn." Emphasis on environmental relationships reminds you that antecedents (what happens before) and consequences (what happens after) can increase or decrease the likelihood of behaviors in the future. Data-based decision-making means that supervisors use the information you collect—frequency counts, durations, percentages—to evaluate whether current plans are working and whether changes are needed. The exam expects you to recognize this logic when choosing between options like "guess what to do" versus "follow the plan and collect data."

1.3 The RBT's Role on the ABA Team

THE RBT IS THE "FRONTLINE implementer" of ABA services. You are typically the person who spends the most direct time with clients, runs teaching programs, and implements behavior-reduction strategies as written by your supervisor. At the same time, your role is clearly limited: you do not design or independently modify treatment plans.

Typical RBT responsibilities:

- Implement written skill-acquisition and behavior-reduction plans
- Collect accurate, reliable data during sessions
- Communicate observations and concerns to your supervisor

Implementing written plans means you follow the instructions your supervisor has provided about prompts, reinforcement, consequences, and how to respond to specific behaviors. You do not "freestyle" major changes, even if you think another approach might work better; any changes must go through your supervisor. Collecting accurate data is central because supervisors depend on your records to make treatment decisions; if your data are incomplete or inaccurate, the team may reach the wrong conclusions about progress. Communication with your supervisor includes reporting significant changes in behavior, injuries, suspected abuse or neglect, and any factors that might affect safety or treatment, always within the limits of your scope and training.

1.4 Where RBTs Work and What Stays the Same

RBTS WORK IN A VARIETY of settings: clinics, homes, schools, and community locations such as parks, stores, or job sites. Each setting brings its own routines, distractions, and practical challenges. Despite those differences, the core expectations for RBT behavior remain the same across environments.

Common service settings and constants:

- Clinics, homes, schools, and community environments
- Consistent expectations for following plans and collecting data
- Ongoing focus on safety, dignity, and professionalism

In clinics, you may have structured schedules, multiple technicians, and quick access to supervisors, but you still must run programs as written and document sessions carefully. In homes and community settings, routines can be less predictable and family preferences may influence how sessions look, yet you are still responsible for following the treatment plan, protecting confidentiality, and maintaining professional boundaries. School settings add coordination with teachers and other staff, requiring clear communication about goals and strategies while respecting school rules and schedules. Across all these environments, your responsibility to follow the plan, keep clients safe, collect accurate data, and uphold the RBT Ethics Code does not change, and exam scenarios often test whether you hold this line under real-world pressures.

1.5 Supervision, Scope of Practice, and Ethics

RBTS MUST WORK UNDER ongoing supervision that meets BACB requirements. Your supervisor is accountable for the clinical direction of services, and you are accountable for implementing what they design. Ethics and scope of practice questions on the exam frequently test whether you know when to act independently and when to involve your supervisor.

Key supervision and ethics themes:

- You do not practice independently as an RBT
- Serious issues are reported promptly to your supervisor
- The RBT Ethics Code guides everyday decisions

Not practicing independently means you should never provide ABA services without an assigned qualified supervisor and should not advertise yourself as an independent clinician. When serious issues occur—such as injuries, abrupt changes in behavior, suspected abuse, or requests to change treatment from parents or teachers—you document accurately and contact your supervisor instead of making major decisions alone. The RBT Ethics Code requires you to protect client rights, respect confidentiality, avoid dual relationships and conflicts of interest, and stay within your competence level. On exam questions, options that ignore supervision, stretch your role, or violate ethical guidelines are almost always incorrect, even if they seem to "solve" a short-term problem.

1.6 Core ABA Vocabulary: Behavior, A–B–C, and Consequences

CERTAIN ABA TERMS APPEAR everywhere in the RBT world and on the exam. Understanding them in simple, practical language will help you decode scenario-based questions quickly. These core words describe how behavior is observed, recorded, and understood in relation to its context.

Essential terms to recognize:

- Behavior as observable, measurable action
- Antecedent–Behavior–Consequence (A-B-C) sequence
- Consequences that increase or decrease behavior

Behavior in ABA means anything a person does that can be observed and measured: walking, screaming, writing, pointing, or completing a puzzle. The A-B-C sequence summarizes how you look at behavior: you note what happens immediately before (antecedent), what the behavior itself is, and what happens immediately after (consequence). Consequences are not "good" or "bad" in a moral sense; they are events that may increase (reinforce) or decrease (punish) the likelihood of the behavior in the future. Exam questions frequently describe a short A-B-C pattern and ask what is happening or what the RBT should do next, so being fluent with this vocabulary is crucial for accurate, quick reasoning.

1.7 Reinforcement, Punishment, and Function (High-Level)

REINFORCEMENT AND PUNISHMENT describe how consequences affect future behavior. The same event can be reinforcing for one person and neutral or punishing for another, so you must pay attention to what actually happens to behavior over time. Function adds another layer by asking why a behavior is happening—what outcome it produces for the learner.

High-level consequences and functions:

- Reinforcement increases the future likelihood of a behavior
- Punishment decreases the future likelihood of a behavior
- Behaviors often serve functions such as attention, tangibles, escape, or automatic (sensory)

Reinforcement can be positive (something added after the behavior, such as praise or access to a toy) or negative (something unpleasant removed, such as ending a task), but in both cases the key feature is that the behavior happens more often in similar situations. Punishment, by contrast, refers to consequences after which the behavior decreases in the future; RBTs follow written plans and ethical guidelines carefully when implementing any procedures that could function as punishment. Functional thinking focuses on what the behavior accomplishes: does it get attention, access to items, escape from demands, or internal sensory effects? On the exam, you are not expected to conduct functional analyses, but you are expected to follow the written plan based on identified function and to avoid accidentally reinforcing problem behavior by, for example, allowing easy escape from tasks when the plan says otherwise.

1.8 Safety, Dignity, and Professional Conduct

CLIENT SAFETY AND DIGNITY are non-negotiable. As an RBT, you are often the person closest to the client when something unexpected happens, so you must act calmly, follow safety procedures, and respect the client as a person at all times. Professional conduct is not just about big ethical violations; it also covers everyday interactions, communication, and boundaries.

Safety and professionalism essentials:

- Protect physical safety and follow crisis and emergency procedures
- Maintain client dignity and confidentiality in all settings
- Avoid dual relationships and conflicts of interest

Protecting safety means following agency procedures for emergencies, using approved crisis strategies if they are part of the plan and you are trained, and reporting injuries or serious incidents promptly. Maintaining dignity includes speaking respectfully about clients, avoiding sarcasm or ridicule, and making reasonable efforts to provide privacy during personal care or sensitive tasks. Confidentiality requires you to protect identifying information, avoid discussing clients in public spaces, and never post about clients on social media, even without names or photos. Avoiding dual relationships means you do not take on roles such as babysitter, roommate, or close friend with clients or their families, and you are cautious about accepting gifts or favors that could impact your professional judgment; these themes show up frequently in ethics-style exam questions.

1.9 How the Exam Uses Scenarios to Test Fundamentals

MOST RBT EXAM QUESTIONS are short scenarios, not pure definition items. Instead of asking you to recite a term, they describe a situation and ask what an RBT should do next or which option is most ethical. Many of these scenarios rely on the basic ideas in this chapter, especially behavior definitions, A-B-C relations, function, and scope of practice.

Typical scenario patterns:

- Choosing actions that match your role and supervision
- Applying simple A-B-C and function logic
- Checking for ethics and client rights in each option

When a question asks what to do in response to a sudden behavior change or a parent request, the exam is really checking whether you will collect data, follow the plan, and contact your supervisor instead of improvising major changes. When a question presents a short A-B-C sequence, you often need to identify whether behavior is being reinforced or punished, or which function is most likely involved at a very basic level. Ethics is woven throughout: you should discard answers that involve sharing private information casually, ignoring clear safety issues, or acting outside your training even if those answers seem faster or easier. Thinking in these patterns will help you navigate many different question types effectively.

1.10 Study Strategies for This Chapter

FUNDAMENTALS ARE EASIER to remember when you connect them to real people and sessions instead of memorizing definitions in isolation. This chapter covers a lot of vocabulary and role boundaries, but they all point back to the same core tasks: follow the plan, take data, protect clients, and communicate appropriately with your supervisor. Good study habits now will pay off in later chapters where these ideas reappear in more specific forms.

Practical study moves:

- Build a small glossary in your own words

- Practice labeling A-B-C and possible functions in everyday situations
- Review supervision, ethics, and role boundaries with your supervisor or trainer

Building a personal glossary means writing each key term—behavior, antecedent, consequence, reinforcement, punishment, function—in your own simple language with one or two concrete examples. Practicing A-B-C with everyday events (for example, "phone buzzes – check phone – notification disappears") helps you see how these concepts apply outside formal sessions, making them easier to recognize on the exam. Reviewing supervision and ethics expectations with your supervisor clarifies what you are and are not allowed to do, and those clarifications will often match the "right answer" pattern in ethical scenarios. By returning to this chapter as you progress, you reinforce a consistent mental model of what an RBT is supposed to do in both routine and challenging situations.

Practice Questions – Chapter 1: RBT Exam and Fundamentals

CHOOSE THE **best** answer for each question.

1. The primary purpose of the RBT certification is to:
   A. Prepare individuals to act as independent behavior analysts
   B. Verify entry-level competence in implementing behavior-analytic services
   C. Allow technicians to diagnose mental disorders
   D. Certify supervisors for other RBTs
2. Which statement best describes the RBT exam?
   A. An essay-based test focused on treatment planning
   B. A computer-based multiple-choice test based on the RBT Task List
   C. An oral interview with a BCBA
   D. A performance-only evaluation with no written portion
3. Which activity is **most** consistent with the RBT role?
   A. Writing new intervention plans for each client
   B. Implementing programs and collecting data under supervision
   C. Approving treatment plans for insurance reimbursement
   D. Discharging clients from services
4. An RBT is unsure how to run a new teaching program that was added to the plan. What is the **best** action?
   A. Make up a similar program that seems right
   B. Skip the program until the next staff meeting
   C. Ask the supervisor for clarification or additional training
   D. Ask the parent how they think it should be done
5. Which of the following is the best example of behavior in ABA terms?
   A. "Being disrespectful"
   B. "Having a bad attitude"
   C. "Saying 'no' and walking away from the table"
   D. "Having ADHD"
6. In the A-B-C sequence, the **consequence** is:
   A. What happens before the behavior
   B. The function of the behavior
   C. What happens after the behavior
   D. The topography of the behavior

7. A learner claps their hands. The therapist immediately gives praise and a sticker, and hand clapping increases in the future. The sticker and praise are:
   A. Punishers
   B. Reinforcers
   C. Antecedents
   D. Baselines
8. Which statement about reinforcement is **most accurate**?
   A. It always involves giving a tangible item
   B. It only works if the person says they like it
   C. It is defined by its effect on future behavior
   D. It must happen on a fixed schedule
9. A student throws materials off the desk. The teacher removes the worksheet, and as a result, this behavior happens more often in the future when work is given. The behavior is most likely:
   A. Positively reinforced by teacher attention
   B. Negatively reinforced by escape from work
   C. Punished by removal of materials
   D. Unrelated to consequences
10. Which situation best represents behavior maintained by **tangible** reinforcement?
    A. A learner screams until they receive a favorite toy
    B. A learner makes jokes so peers laugh
    C. A learner pinches themselves because it feels stimulating
    D. A learner puts their head down to avoid classwork
11. Which of the following best describes the RBT's relationship with a supervisor?
    A. The RBT and supervisor share equal responsibility for clinical decisions
    B. The supervisor designs the programs and the RBT implements them
    C. The RBT supervises other technicians and reports to the supervisor monthly
    D. The RBT can ignore the supervisor's feedback if experienced
12. An RBT notices that a client has bruises that were not there in the previous session, and the client seems fearful. What is the **best** first step?
    A. Ignore the bruises because they might be an accident
    B. Take photos and post them in a staff social media group
    C. Document what was observed and report it according to agency and supervisor guidance
    D. Question the caregiver aggressively at pickup
13. Which statement best reflects **scope of practice** for an RBT?
    A. RBTs can provide ABA services independently if they feel confident
    B. RBTs can design treatment plans if the BCBA is busy
    C. RBTs must work under ongoing supervision and stay within tasks they are trained and authorized to do
    D. RBTs can provide counseling and mental health therapy when needed
14. Maintaining client dignity includes:
    A. Using nicknames and jokes about the client during staff meetings
    B. Ensuring privacy when possible during personal care or sensitive activities
    C. Sharing funny stories about the client with friends as long as no names are used
    D. Ignoring the client when they attempt to communicate
15. Which action is **most likely** a violation of confidentiality?

A. Discussing client progress with your BCBA supervisor
B. Sharing data with a teacher who is on the treatment team
C. Talking about a client's behavior in a crowded elevator using their first name
D. Writing a session note in the secure electronic health record

16. An RBT works in a school, a clinic, and in the community with the same client. Which statement is **most accurate**?
A. The RBT should use different treatment plans in each setting based on what feels right
B. The RBT's core responsibilities—following plans, taking data, protecting dignity—stay the same across settings
C. Ethics only apply in the clinic because it is a health-care setting
D. Confidentiality does not apply when working in schools

17. A parent offers the RBT expensive concert tickets as a "thank you." What is the **best** response?
A. Accept the tickets but do not tell anyone
B. Accept and post a thank-you message with the parent's name
C. Politely decline and explain agency or ethical guidelines about gifts, then inform the supervisor
D. Accept the tickets if the parent insists

18. Which scenario best reflects **appropriate** professional boundaries for an RBT?
A. Babysitting for the client on weekends for extra income
B. Becoming the client's social media friend to "stay connected"
C. Interacting with the client only in professional contexts and following agency policies
D. Inviting the client's family to personal parties

19. Which statement about the RBT exam format is true?
A. It is open-note and open-book
B. It includes multiple-choice questions with a fixed time limit
C. It uses short-answer questions but no multiple-choice
D. It can be taken without prior training or supervision requirements

20. Why does the exam use many scenario-based questions?
A. To check if you have memorized definitions word for word
B. To see if you can apply fundamentals and ethics to realistic situations
C. To test advanced research design skills
D. To assess your writing ability

21. An RBT notices that a client's aggressive behavior suddenly increases and is more intense than usual. What should the RBT do **first**?
A. Stop all current programs and start new ones
B. Document the behavior carefully and notify the supervisor promptly
C. Call the client's doctor to recommend medication
D. Ignore the change until the next scheduled supervision meeting

22. Which of the following is the **best** high-level definition of ABA for an RBT?
A. A method for controlling people
B. A science focused on understanding and improving socially significant behavior using behavioral principles
C. A type of counseling that focuses on emotions
D. A medical approach that prescribes medication

23. An RBT is asked by a friend, "What do you actually do as an RBT?" Which response best reflects the role?
A. "I diagnose behavior disorders and prescribe treatment."

B. "I design and approve all the treatment plans."
C. "I work directly with clients to run programs and collect data that my supervisor uses to guide treatment."
D. "I manage the entire clinic by myself."

24. A new RBT is trying to remember terms like behavior, antecedent, consequence, and function. Which study approach is **most consistent** with this chapter's suggestions?
    A. Reading the definitions once and hoping to remember them
    B. Creating a small glossary in their own words with everyday examples
    C. Only studying the night before the exam
    D. Ignoring these terms and focusing only on ethics
25. Why is it important for RBTs to understand functions of behavior at a basic level, even if they do not design plans?
    A. It allows them to conduct independent functional analyses
    B. It helps them choose new interventions without supervision
    C. It helps them appreciate why the written plan emphasizes certain responses and avoid accidentally reinforcing problem behavior
    D. It is only necessary for passing the exam and not for actual work

Answer Key – Chapter 1 (With Justifications)

1. **B** – The RBT certification verifies **entry-level competence** in implementing ABA services under supervision, not independent clinical practice or supervision of others.
2. **B** – The RBT exam is a **computer-based multiple-choice test** built around the RBT Task List and related requirements, not essays or oral interviews.
3. **B** – Implementing programs and collecting data under the direction of a qualified supervisor is central to the RBT role; writing or approving plans is outside typical scope.
4. **C** – When unsure how to implement a program, the RBT should **seek clarification or training from the supervisor**, not improvise or ignore parts of the plan.
5. **C** – "Saying 'no' and walking away from the table" is specific, observable, and measurable, matching the ABA definition of behavior better than labels or diagnoses.
6. **C** – The **consequence** is what happens immediately **after** the behavior, which can influence whether the behavior is more or less likely in the future.
7. **B** – Because hand clapping **increases** in the future after stickers and praise, those events function as **reinforcers** for that behavior.
8. **C** – Reinforcement is defined by its effect: it is any consequence that **increases the future likelihood** of a behavior, regardless of whether it seems pleasant.
9. **B** – Removing the worksheet after the behavior and then seeing that behavior increase suggests **negative reinforcement by escape** from work.
10. **A** – Screaming that continues until a favorite toy is delivered is most consistent with behavior maintained by **tangible** reinforcement (access to items).
11. **B** – The supervisor designs and oversees treatment; the RBT **implements** those plans and collects data, working under supervision rather than as an equal clinical decision-maker.
12. **C** – The RBT should **document objectively** and follow reporting procedures (including informing the supervisor) rather than ignoring, posting publicly, or confronting inappropriately.
13. **C** – RBTs must **work under supervision** and keep to the tasks for which they are trained and authorized;

designing or independently delivering services is outside their scope.

14. **B** – Protecting dignity includes **respecting privacy** and avoiding unnecessary embarrassment or humiliation, especially during personal or sensitive situations.
15. C – Talking about a client's behavior in a crowded elevator using their first name risks exposing identifiable information and violates **confidentiality** expectations.
16. **B** – While settings differ, the RBT's core duties—**following plans, collecting data, upholding ethics and confidentiality**—remain the same across environments.
17. C – Accepting large gifts can create conflicts of interest; the RBT should **politely decline**, explain policies, and inform the supervisor.
18. C – Keeping the relationship strictly **professional and policy-consistent** demonstrates appropriate boundaries; babysitting, social media friendships, and party invitations blur those lines.
19. **B** – The exam consists of **multiple-choice questions** with a time limit; it is not open-book and still requires meeting training and supervision prerequisites.
20. **B** – Scenario-based questions assess whether you can **apply fundamentals and ethics** in realistic situations, not just memorize definitions.
21. **B** – The RBT should **document carefully and contact the supervisor**, rather than ignoring the change or independently altering treatment or making medical recommendations.
22. **B** – ABA is a **science** that focuses on understanding and improving socially significant behavior using behavioral principles and data-based decisions.
23. C – This response correctly states that the RBT **works directly with clients** implementing programs and collecting data that supervisors use to guide treatment.
24. **B** – Building a **glossary in your own words with everyday examples** aligns with recommendations to make terms meaningful and easier to remember.
25. C – Understanding behavior functions helps RBTs see **why** plans are written a certain way and avoid accidentally reinforcing problem behavior, even though they do not design the plans themselves.

Chapter 2: Professionalism, Ethics, and Scope of Practice

Professionalism and ethics are at the core of your work as an RBT. Every session, note, conversation, and decision is shaped by rules about how you treat clients, families, coworkers, and supervisors. This chapter turns those expectations into clear behaviors you can recognize in exam scenarios and in real life. When you can quickly spot what is ethical, within scope, and professional, many "tricky" exam questions become much easier to answer.

2.1 Why Professionalism Matters for RBTs

PROFESSIONALISM IS more than being polite or wearing a name badge. It is the consistent way you respect clients and families, follow plans and procedures, and represent your supervisor and organization. As the person who often spends the most time with the client, you are the face of ABA for many families.

Core professionalism themes:

- Reliability and follow-through
- Respectful communication
- Representing your role and organization accurately

Reliability and follow-through mean you show up on time, prepared, and ready to work the entire scheduled session. You complete required paperwork and data collection promptly, not days later when details are fuzzy. When you are sick or running late, you follow your organization's procedures for notifying the right person as soon as possible. On exam questions, an RBT who frequently cancels, arrives late without notice, or ignores documentation responsibilities is rarely portrayed as acting professionally. Professional answers tend to show the RBT honoring commitments and handling unavoidable changes responsibly.

Respectful communication includes how you speak to and about clients, families, teachers, and coworkers. You use calm, neutral, and non-judgmental language even when describing challenging behavior or difficult days. You avoid sarcasm, teasing, or gossip and take care not to blame clients or families in your words. When conflicts or misunderstandings occur, you respond with patience and curiosity instead of anger or disrespect. In exam scenarios, answers that highlight clear, respectful communication almost always beat those that show frustration or rudeness.

Representing your role and organization accurately means you do not speak or act as if you are the BCBA or decision-maker when you are not. You explain that your job is to implement the behavior plan and collect data under supervision, not to design treatment or change services on your own. You avoid making promises about goals, hours, or timelines that only your supervisor or organization can approve. When families or staff ask questions outside your role, you give basic information and then direct them to your supervisor for final answers. On the exam, the correct choice is usually the one where the RBT stays honest about their role and does not overstep.

2.2 The RBT Ethics Code in Everyday Language

THE RBT ETHICS CODE gives concrete rules about what you must and must not do as an RBT. You are not expected to memorize the code numbers, but you are expected to understand what ethical behavior looks like in common situations. Many exam items describe a short scenario and expect you to pick the response that best fits the spirit of the Ethics Code.

Big ethics code ideas:

- Protect client welfare, rights, and dignity
- Work under supervision and within your competence
- Be honest and follow laws, regulations, and policies

Protecting client welfare, rights, and dignity means that client well-being comes before convenience, pressure, or personal feelings. You avoid doing anything that could harm or humiliate a client, even if someone else suggests it or says "we've always done it this way." When you see something that seems unsafe or disrespectful, you do not ignore it; you bring it to your supervisor. On exam questions, options that prioritize client safety and respect are almost always correct compared to options that save time or please others but risk harm.

Working under supervision and within your competence reminds you that the RBT role is supervised and limited. You do not present yourself as a behavior analyst, therapist, or counselor who can diagnose or design treatment independently. When given a task you do not understand or have not been trained to do, you say so and request training or clarification. You implement only those procedures that your supervisor has authorized and that you feel competent to perform safely. The exam frequently tests whether the RBT knows when to stop and asks for help instead of guessing.

Being honest and following laws, regulations, and policies includes truthfulness in documentation, billing, and communication. You never change data to "look better," record sessions that did not happen, or sign forms you know are inaccurate. You follow rules about privacy, mandated reporting, and safety, even when it feels inconvenient. When a mistake occurs, you report it honestly and work with your supervisor to correct it instead of hiding it. Exam answers that involve falsifying data, bending rules, or lying are clear ethics violations and should be avoided.

2.3 Client Rights, Dignity, and Assent

CLIENTS HAVE RIGHTS that do not disappear just because they receive ABA services. They have the right to be treated respectfully, to have their privacy protected, and, when possible, to have a say in what happens to them. Even clients with limited communication skills can show assent or protest through their behavior, and you are expected to notice these signals.

Dignity and rights in practice:

- Use respectful language and protect privacy
- Offer reasonable choices and honor preferences when possible
- Attend to assent, protest, and signs of distress

Using respectful language and protecting privacy means you avoid negative labels like "manipulative," "lazy," or "noncompliant" when talking about a client. You describe what you see behaviorally and keep personal details out of public spaces, like hallways and waiting rooms. You avoid discussing client stories with friends, family, or strangers, even if you omit names. You also do not post about clients on social media under any circumstances. On the exam, actions that keep personal information private and maintain neutral, respectful wording indicate ethically sound behavior.

Offering reasonable choices and honoring preferences when possible helps clients feel respected and increases cooperation. You might let the client choose which task to do first, which reinforcer to work for, or where to sit, as long as these options fit within the plan. You do not promise choices that violate the behavior plan or safety rules, but you do use choice-making as a tool for dignity and engagement. In exam scenarios, the better answers often include simple, appropriate choices rather than strict control over every detail.

Attending to assent, protest, and signs of distress means you watch how the client responds to activities, demands, and settings. If the client clearly shows fear, pain, or repeated strong resistance, you still follow the plan but also document and report these reactions to your supervisor. You may use strategies like breaks, pairing, and adjustments allowed by the plan to reduce distress. You do not ignore ongoing signs that a client is deeply uncomfortable or overwhelmed. On the test, ignoring obvious distress without informing the supervisor or checking the plan is rarely the correct choice.

2.4 Confidentiality and Protecting Information

CONFIDENTIALITY MEANS keeping client information private and secure. As an RBT, you regularly see and hear sensitive details about diagnoses, family situations, locations, and behavior. You are responsible for making sure those details are only shared with people who are allowed to know and in ways that meet legal and organizational rules.

Confidentiality basics:

- Share information only with authorized people who need to know
- Avoid discussing clients in public or online
- Store and transmit data securely and according to policy

Sharing information only with authorized people who need to know means you talk about clients with your supervisor, your clinical team, and other approved professionals involved in the case. You do not share details with friends, extended family, neighbors, or other staff who are not on the case. Even with authorized people, you share information that is relevant to treatment, not gossip. On exam questions, the safe answers limit sharing to the professional circle with a legitimate reason to know.

Avoiding discussion of clients in public or online means you do not talk about them in places where others can easily overhear, such as lobbies, hallways, elevators, or social events. You never post stories, screenshots, or photos from sessions on social media, even if you think they are anonymous. You also avoid using messages or group chats that are not approved for confidential communication. The exam often presents situations where an RBT "just tells a friend" or posts a "funny story" online, and these are clear confidentiality violations.

Storing and transmitting data securely and according to policy means you use the systems and procedures your organization has set up for privacy. Paper notes are locked away when not in use, and electronic records are entered in secure platforms using your own login. You do not leave session notes in your car or on a kitchen table where others can read them. You do not take photos or videos on personal devices unless your organization and supervisor explicitly authorize and manage that process. On exam items, correct answers favor secure, policy-compliant handling of data over informal or convenient shortcuts.

2.5 Boundaries, Dual Relationships, and Gifts

BOUNDARIES KEEP YOUR role as a professional clear and protect both you and the client from conflicts of interest. Because RBTs spend a lot of time with families, it can be tempting to drift into more personal roles, but the Ethics Code requires you to avoid dual relationships and inappropriate gifts.

Boundary red flags:

- Mixing professional and personal roles
- Accepting significant gifts or favors
- Oversharing or socializing beyond professional limits

Mixing professional and personal roles happens when you become a babysitter, family friend, roommate, or romantic partner with a client or their family. Even if everyone is friendly and well-intentioned, these relationships can make it hard to be objective and can influence decisions about services. A dual relationship can also make it harder for clients and families to say "no" to your requests or disagree with your work. On exam questions, the RBT should politely decline invitations that clearly cross into personal roles and discuss boundary concerns with their supervisor.

Accepting significant gifts or favors can create a sense of obligation and may look like favoritism or an attempt to influence your behavior. While some agencies allow small, low-value tokens (like a small holiday treat), expensive or repeated gifts are usually not appropriate. If a family offers something that feels more than a small thank-you, the ethical response is to decline and explain your organization's policy. On the exam, answers where the RBT quietly accepts large gifts or trades favors usually signal unethical behavior.

Oversharing or socializing beyond professional limits includes telling families too much about your personal life or meeting them socially outside of work for non-treatment reasons. You can be warm and genuine without sharing private details about your relationships, finances, or problems. Likewise, you do not send personal social media requests, enter group chats with clients, or text them about non-work topics. In test scenarios, the RBT who keeps communication focused on treatment and stays off personal channels is typically portrayed as acting ethically.

2.6 Cultural Responsiveness and Respecting Differences

RBTS WORK WITH PEOPLE from many cultural, linguistic, and religious backgrounds. Professionalism includes approaching these differences with respect and curiosity instead of assumptions or judgment. When families feel that their culture is valued, they are more likely to stay engaged in treatment and share important information with the team.

Culturally responsive behavior:

- Listening and asking respectful questions about family preferences
- Avoiding stereotypes and biased comments
- Working with your supervisor to adapt within ethical and clinical limits

Listening and asking respectful questions means you explore what matters to the family, such as daily routines, dress, food, holidays, and expectations for behavior at home. If something in the plan seems to conflict with a cultural or religious practice, you do not dismiss it as "weird" or "wrong." Instead, you ask how the family sees it and share that information with your supervisor. On exam questions, the RBT who listens and checks rather than assuming is usually the one acting professionally.

Avoiding stereotypes and biased comments means you never treat clients or families in a certain way "because people from that group are always like this." You do not make jokes, remarks, or generalizations about race, language, religion, or culture. You evaluate behavior and progress based on individual data, not group assumptions. Test items that include stereotyping, mocking, or disrespectful opinions about culture are clearly unethical and should not be chosen.

Working with your supervisor to adapt within ethical and clinical limits means you do not personally rewrite treatment to match every preference, but you also do not ignore genuine cultural concerns. If a family's values conflict with some part of the plan, you explain that you must follow the current plan and then share their concerns with your supervisor. Together, your supervisory team may decide to adjust procedures or goals. In exam scenarios, the correct answer often includes both respect for culture and respect for the chain of supervision.

2.7 Scope of Practice vs. Scope of Competence

SCOPE OF PRACTICE REFERS to what the RBT role in general is allowed to do. Scope of competence is about what you personally have been trained and can do safely and correctly. Ethical practice requires you to stay within both: you do not take on tasks that are outside the RBT role, and you do not perform tasks within the role if you do not yet know how.

Staying in-bounds:

- Implement written plans; do not design or majorly change them
- Decline tasks you are not trained for and request training
- Do not advertise or deliver independent ABA services

Implementing written plans and not designing or majorly changing them means you follow the programs, behavior plans, and procedures created by your supervisor. You can make small choices within the plan (like which reinforcer to try first) but you do not decide to stop using reinforcement or add a new consequence without approval. When parents, teachers, or others request changes, you explain your role and offer to connect them with your supervisor. On the exam, RBTs who rewrite treatment plans alone are routinely shown as exceeding their scope.

Declining tasks you are not trained for and requesting training shows that you understand your responsibility for safe implementation. If you're asked to use a new restraint, crisis procedure, or data system you have never learned, you say that you need proper training first. You do not guess or "wing it," especially when safety is involved. In test items, the RBT who acknowledges their limits and seeks supervision is generally doing the right thing.

Not advertising or delivering independent ABA services means you do not use your RBT credential to provide unsupervised "side" services in homes, schools, or online. The RBT credential assumes you are working under a responsible certificant or qualified supervisor through an organization or arrangement that meets BACB requirements. Offering freelance ABA on your own, especially to your current clients, violates both supervision and scope rules. Exam answers that involve "off-the-books" sessions or independent work should be avoided.

2.8 Supervision, Feedback, and Professional Growth

SUPERVISION IS NOT just a formality; it is part of what makes ABA services safe, ethical, and effective. RBTs are required to receive a certain amount of supervision, but the quality of that supervision depends partly on how you participate. Good RBTs are active learners who seek feedback and share relevant information instead of hiding it.

Healthy supervision habits:

- Maintain regular, documented contact with your supervisor
- Communicate openly about cases, data, and challenges
- Accept feedback and use it to improve

Maintaining regular, documented contact means you know who your supervisor is and you meet or connect according to BACB and organizational requirements. Some of that supervision time must include your supervisor directly observing your work with clients. You attend scheduled meetings, respond to messages, and provide data or updates when requested. On exam questions, an RBT who never meets with a supervisor or does not know who supervises them is clearly not following expectations.

Communicating openly about cases, data, and challenges means you share accurate information rather than hiding errors or problems. If a procedure is not working, data is missing, a family is frequently cancelling, or an incident occurs, you let your supervisor know. You do not change data to make things look better or keep serious concerns to yourself. In exam scenarios, the more ethical answer is the one where the RBT is honest, even if it feels uncomfortable.

Accepting feedback and using it to improve means you understand that feedback is a normal and important part of the job. You listen carefully, ask questions if you are confused, and practice what your supervisor suggests. Even if feedback is hard to hear, you respond professionally instead of arguing or refusing. The exam often shows RBTs who either embrace feedback or reject it; the one who works with feedback is typically the correct model.

2.9 Handling Concerns, Incidents, and Suspected Abuse

SOMETIMES YOU WILL see things that are serious: injuries, sudden changes in behavior, unsafe environments, or possible signs of abuse or neglect. As an RBT, you must respond in a way that protects the client and follows legal and organizational rules. The exam frequently asks what you should do first when something concerning happens.

When something is wrong:

- Act to ensure immediate safety when there is urgent risk
- Document events objectively and notify your supervisor

- Follow mandated reporting and agency procedures

Acting to ensure immediate safety when there is urgent risk means you use the crisis or emergency procedures you have been trained on. If a client is in danger of serious harm right now, you may need to remove dangerous items, move other people away, or call emergency services according to your agency's plan. You do not ignore a dangerous situation because you are afraid of causing trouble. In exam questions, responses that protect immediate safety are favored over those that delay action.

Documenting events objectively and notifying your supervisor means you write down exactly what you saw or heard, without guessing motives or assigning blame. You include details like time, place, and specific behaviors or statements, then contact your supervisor promptly using the approved method. You do not wait until the next monthly meeting or casually mention it in passing. The pattern "document and inform your supervisor" appears regularly in exam answers for serious but not life-threatening issues.

Following mandated reporting and agency procedures may be required by law, especially in cases of suspected abuse, neglect, or exploitation. Your organization should train you on how to respond if you suspect abuse, including whether you are a mandated reporter and how to file a report. You work with your supervisor and follow those steps even if you are unsure how others will react. On test items, answers that keep serious concerns "secret" or handled only within the family are usually incorrect.

2.10 How the Exam Tests Professionalism and Ethics

THE RBT EXAM DOES NOT usually ask you to name specific Ethics Code sections. Instead, it tests your ability to spot ethical and unethical behavior in short stories about parents, staff, social media, gifts, and supervision. If you know what "good RBT behavior" looks like, many questions will feel predictable.

Common exam patterns:

- Temptations to exceed your scope or ignore supervision
- Scenarios with confidentiality, dignity, or boundary violations
- Correct options that protect client rights and follow the plan

Temptations to exceed your scope or ignore supervision often look helpful at first glance. The scenario may show an RBT who wants to design a new plan, agree to a parent's request that conflicts with the plan, or make a diagnosis to calm a worried teacher. These answers feel active, but they are not appropriate for an RBT. Correct answers usually include some version of "follow the plan" and "talk to your supervisor" instead of "fix it alone."

Scenarios with confidentiality, dignity, or boundary violations might include posting about clients online, accepting large gifts, discussing clients publicly, or treating clients in a disrespectful way. Often, everyone around the RBT in the story is acting casually or unprofessionally to make it tempting to join in. On the exam, the correct answer is the one where the RBT chooses not to participate and, when needed, reports the concern through proper channels.

Correct options that protect client rights and follow the plan usually involve maintaining privacy, using respectful language, upholding consent and cultural respect, and staying within your role. When two answers look reasonable, ask yourself which one better protects the client's safety, dignity, and confidentiality while honoring supervision. In most ethics and professionalism questions, that will point you to the right choice.

Practice Questions – Chapter 2 (Professionalism, Ethics, Scope)

CHOOSE THE **best** answer for each question.

1. A parent asks you to use a punishment procedure they saw online that is **not** part of the behavior plan. What should you do first?

A. Try it in the next session to see if it works
B. Use it only when the BCBA is not present
C. Explain that you must follow the written plan and inform your supervisor about the parent's request
D. Add the procedure to the plan yourself and tell the BCBA later

2. Which situation is the **best** example of maintaining client dignity?
A. Discussing a client's embarrassing behavior loudly in the lobby
B. Making jokes about a client's stimming with coworkers
C. Providing privacy during toileting and using neutral, respectful language in documentation
D. Secretly recording sessions and sharing them with friends

3. An RBT is invited to a client's birthday party outside of work hours. What is the **most appropriate** response?
A. Accept the invitation and stay all day
B. Politely decline and explain the need to maintain professional boundaries
C. Attend but avoid talking to the client's parents
D. Attend only if the BCBA goes too

4. During a session, you see several fresh bruises on a child's arm and they flinch when an adult approaches. What should you do?
A. Ignore it because you do not want to overreact
B. Post about it in a private group chat with coworkers
C. Document your observations objectively and follow your agency's and supervisor's reporting procedures
D. Accuse the caregiver of abuse in front of the child

5. Which task is clearly **outside** an RBT's scope of practice?
A. Implementing a behavior plan written by a BCBA
B. Collecting frequency data on a target behavior
C. Diagnosing autism and creating a treatment plan
D. Reporting a safety concern to a supervisor

6. A parent offers you a $200 gift card to thank you for your work. Your agency policy allows only small, token gifts. What should you do?
A. Accept it and keep it secret
B. Accept it and post a thank-you message on social media
C. Politely decline, explain the policy, and let your supervisor know
D. Accept it but reduce reinforcement for the client to appear fair

7. Which of the following best protects client confidentiality?
A. Talking about a client's behavior in a coffee shop using only their first name
B. Sharing detailed stories with a friend who is "also in health care"
C. Discussing cases only with authorized team members and keeping records in secure systems
D. Texting session details to friends to get their opinion

8. A teacher asks you to "stop using reinforcers" because they think it is bribery, even though the BCBA's plan includes reinforcement. What is the best response?
A. Stop using reinforcers to keep the teacher happy
B. Explain that you must follow the BCBA's plan and offer to connect the teacher with your supervisor
C. Use reinforcers only when the teacher is not watching
D. Change the plan yourself so it no longer uses reinforcement

9. Which scenario best describes a **dual relationship**?
A. Working with a client at home and in the community

B. Being supervised by more than one BCBA
C. Serving as the client's RBT and being their paid babysitter on weekends
D. Consulting with a school team about the same client

10. An RBT "rounds up" data to make it look like a client is improving faster. Which statement is most accurate?
A. This is acceptable if the parent wants to see progress
B. This is acceptable if the BCBA is very busy
C. This is unethical because it falsifies data used for treatment decisions
D. This is required to keep services approved

11. A family has strong cultural and religious practices that affect their routines. What is the **best** approach for the RBT?
A. Ignore these practices and run sessions the same as with every other family
B. Make jokes about how "strange" their routines are
C. Ask respectful questions, honor reasonable preferences when possible, and share relevant information with the supervisor
D. Tell the family they must change their routines to match the plan

12. A coworker asks to use your login to "quickly update" some client notes. What should you do?
A. Share your login to be helpful
B. Share it but change your password later
C. Refuse to share your login and follow your organization's account security policies
D. Share it only if the coworker is also an RBT

13. Which action best demonstrates appropriate use of supervision?
A. Avoiding meetings because you feel confident on your own
B. Meeting regularly with your supervisor, discussing cases honestly, and asking questions when unsure
C. Sending data to your supervisor only once a year
D. Ignoring feedback that feels uncomfortable

14. A parent asks you for advice about which antidepressant they should take. What is the best response?
A. Share advice based on your personal experience
B. Suggest a medication that worked for another client
C. Explain that this is outside your role and encourage them to talk with a qualified medical provider
D. Look up answers online during the session and read them aloud

15. At a park, another adult points to your client and asks, "Is that child autistic?" What should you do?
A. Confirm the diagnosis and give more details
B. Say "yes" but keep it brief
C. Explain that you cannot share personal information about any client and redirect the conversation
D. Laugh and say you are not allowed to "officially" answer

16. An RBT notices that a coworker frequently yells at clients and uses physical prompts that are not in the plan. What is the best action?
A. Join in so the coworker does not feel judged
B. Ignore it because it is not your job to intervene
C. Document what you observe and report the concern through appropriate supervisory or organizational channels
D. Complain about the coworker to other staff in the break room

17. Which statement best describes **scope of competence** for an RBT?
A. Once you are certified, you can perform any procedure without training

B. You should perform only tasks you have been trained to do competently, even if they are part of the RBT role
C. Competence does not matter if your supervisor is in the building
D. You must accept any assignment your employer gives you

18. A caregiver asks you to reduce the child's hours and "just not tell the BCBA." How should you respond?
A. Secretly end sessions early to help the family
B. Agree as long as you still get paid for full hours
C. Explain that decisions about hours must involve your supervisor and direct the caregiver to speak with them
D. Immediately cut hours and update the plan yourself

19. Which action best reflects appropriate boundaries on social media?
A. Accepting friend requests from clients and families
B. Posting pictures from sessions with emojis over client faces
C. Keeping your personal accounts separate, not connecting with clients or families, and never posting client-related content
D. Messaging clients about their goals through your personal account

20. Your supervisor assigns a new crisis-management procedure and asks if you have been trained. You have not. What should you do?
A. Say nothing and try to figure it out if needed
B. Watch a random video online and then use the procedure
C. Say you have not been trained and request proper training and observation before implementing it
D. Refuse to learn it under any circumstances

21. A parent says a neighbor's RBT does "off-the-books" cash sessions and asks if you will do the same. What is the best response?
A. Agree as long as you are paid in cash
B. Agree but keep it secret from your agency
C. Explain that you can only provide services through your organization under supervision and decline the request
D. Do it once as a favor and then stop

22. Which of the following is the **best** example of objective documentation?
A. "Client was terrible and hates therapy today."
B. "The client is lazy and refuses everything."
C. "Client threw materials 7 times during a 30-minute session when demands were presented."
D. "Client is trying to make staff angry."

23. A client says they "don't want to work with you anymore" and appears upset. What should you do first?
A. Force them to continue so they learn to obey
B. Ignore the comment and keep going as if nothing happened
C. Acknowledge their feelings, continue using supportive strategies within the plan, and inform your supervisor about the situation
D. Threaten to tell their parents if they do not cooperate

24. Which situation best reflects ethical collaboration with other professionals (teachers, therapists, etc.)?
A. Sharing detailed client records with anyone who asks
B. Refusing to talk with teachers at all
C. Sharing relevant information with consent, staying within your role, and involving your supervisor when

appropriate

D. Telling families that other professionals are wrong and your team is right

25. When two answers both seem reasonable on a professionalism/ethics question, which one is **most likely** to be correct?

    A. The one where the RBT changes the plan independently to solve the problem

    B. The one where the RBT acts outside their role to please a parent or teacher

    C. The one where the RBT protects client rights, follows the plan, and contacts the supervisor when needed

    D. The one where the RBT avoids documentation to save time

Answer Key – Chapter 2 (With Justifications)

1. **C** – You must follow the written plan and your supervisor's directions; adding unapproved punishment is outside your role, so you explain this and inform your supervisor.
2. **C** – Providing privacy and using neutral, respectful language supports dignity; joking, public discussion, or secret recordings do not.
3. **B** – Politely declining helps avoid dual relationships and keeps the relationship professional.
4. **C** – You document objectively and follow reporting procedures with your supervisor and agency; ignoring or accusing in front of the child is inappropriate.
5. **C** – Diagnosing and creating treatment plans are not RBT tasks; implementing plans and collecting data are.
6. **C** – Significant gifts can create conflicts of interest; you follow policy by declining and informing your supervisor.
7. **C** – Limiting discussion to authorized team members and using secure systems is the safest way to protect confidentiality.
8. **B** – You must follow the BCBA's plan and direct the teacher's concerns to your supervisor, not change or drop procedures yourself.
9. **C** – Being both the RBT and a paid babysitter mixes professional and personal roles and is a dual relationship.
10. **C** – Changing data to look better is falsification and is unethical because it misleads treatment decisions.
11. **C** – Respectful questions, honoring reasonable preferences, and involving your supervisor when needed show cultural responsiveness and professionalism.
12. **C** – Sharing logins violates security; you must protect your credentials and follow policy.
13. **B** – Regular supervision, open discussion, and questions when unsure match expectations for ethical supervised practice.
14. **C** – Medication advice is outside your role; you direct the parent to a qualified medical professional.
15. **C** – You must protect client information and cannot share diagnoses; a brief, respectful refusal and redirection is appropriate.
16. **C** – Unsafe or unapproved practices should be documented and reported through proper channels to protect clients.
17. **B** – Scope of competence means doing only what you are trained and able to do, even within the broader RBT role.
18. **C** – Decisions about hours belong to the supervisor, caregiver, and possibly the funder; you cannot secretly change hours.
19. **C** – Keeping personal accounts separate and never posting about clients maintains clear online boundaries.
20. **C** – You must be honest about training and ask for proper instruction and observation before using crisis procedures.

21. **C** – Providing unsupervised "off-the-books" services is outside your role; you must decline and explain your limits.
22. **C** – This statement uses clear, observable, and measurable terms without guessing motives, which makes it objective.
23. **C** – You respond with empathy, continue ethically within the plan, and inform your supervisor so they can help address the issue.
24. **C** – Ethical collaboration shares relevant information with consent, respects roles, and involves the supervisor as needed.
25. **C** – The exam favors options where the RBT protects client rights, stays within scope, follows the plan, and uses supervision appropriately.

Chapter 3: Measurement and Assessment

Measurement and assessment are the eyes and ears of ABA. They let your supervisor see what's really happening so they can design, adjust, and evaluate treatment. As an RBT, your main responsibilities are to define behavior clearly, collect accurate data, and participate in basic assessment activities like preference checks and ABC data.

3.1 Why Measurement and Assessment Matter

MEASUREMENT AND ASSESSMENT are the foundation of data-based decision making in ABA. Without them, plans become guesses instead of carefully guided interventions. The RBT exam will expect you to recognize why these processes are essential and what your role is in them.

- They turn behavior into objective, usable information
- They guide treatment decisions and changes
- They support ethical, accountable practice

They turn behavior into objective, usable information by converting "it seemed like a rough day" into numbers and descriptions that can be analyzed. When you tally behaviors, time them, or record ABCs, you give your supervisor data they can graph and interpret. This information shows whether behavior is improving, getting worse, or staying the same. Without those numbers and descriptions, everyone is guessing based on memory and feelings, which can be very inaccurate.

They guide treatment decisions and changes by showing whether current interventions are working. If data show a skill is improving, the supervisor may increase difficulty or start generalization. If data show no progress or worsening behavior, the supervisor may revise goals, prompts, or reinforcement systems. You are not the one making those decisions, but your accurate data directly drive them. On exam questions, the "data-based" option is almost always better than "go with your gut."

They support ethical, accountable practice by creating a record of what you did and what happened. Good measurement and assessment show that services are not random, that behavior changes are real, and that clients are not kept on ineffective plans. If there is ever a question or complaint, clear data and assessment records can demonstrate that decisions were responsible and transparent. The exam often links poor or missing data to ethical red flags such as falsification or low treatment integrity.

3.2 Operational Definitions: Defining What You Measure

AN OPERATIONAL DEFINITION tells everyone exactly what counts as a behavior and what does not. It turns vague labels into specific, observable actions that can be measured reliably. As an RBT, you must understand and follow these definitions when collecting data.

- Use observable and measurable terms
- Include clear examples and non-examples
- Aim for consistency between different observers

Using observable and measurable terms means defining behavior based on what you can see or hear, not on feelings or guesses. Instead of "being disrespectful," a definition might say "raising voice above conversational level and using words such as 'stupid' or 'shut up' toward others." Those words describe exactly what behavior looks and sounds like. On the exam, operational definitions that focus on visible actions beat those that describe attitudes or personality.

Including clear examples and non-examples helps distinguish what should and should not be recorded. For "aggression," examples might include "hitting, kicking, biting, scratching others with enough force to make contact," while non-examples might include "light accidental bumps while walking past someone." This prevents people from counting mild or accidental contact as aggression. Test questions often imply that good definitions outline what is "in" and what is "out" of the category.

Aiming for consistency between different observers is the whole point of defining behavior this way. If two trained RBTs observe the same session using the same definition, they should record similar data. This consistency is sometimes checked through interobserver agreement (IOA). If the definition is vague, agreement will be low because everyone guesses differently. In exam scenarios, definitions that promote agreement are considered higher quality than fuzzy ones that leave room for interpretation.

3.3 Basic Measurement Types: Frequency, Rate, Duration, Latency

ONCE BEHAVIOR IS DEFINED, you need a method for measuring it. Basic measurement types answer questions like "how often," "how long," and "how quickly" behavior happens. The exam frequently asks you to match a behavior description to an appropriate measurement method.

- Frequency and rate for "how often"
- Duration for "how long"
- Latency for "how quickly after a cue"

Frequency and rate for "how often" are used when behavior has a clear start and end and isn't too fast to count. Frequency is a simple count of how many times the behavior occurs, and rate is that count divided by time (like "responses per minute"). Examples include counting hand raises, instances of swearing, or completed tasks. On test questions, if behavior is cleanly countable and the main concern is "how many," frequency or rate are usually the best answer.

Duration for "how long" is used when the length of time a behavior occurs is important. You might time how long a tantrum lasts from the first scream to calm behavior, or how many minutes a learner remains on-task during independent work. Duration can be measured per episode or as total time during a session. When exam items mention goals like "shorter tantrums" or "longer engagement," duration is often the correct measurement choice.

Latency for "how quickly after a cue" measures the time between a prompt and the start of behavior. For example, you might know how long it takes a learner to begin a task after being told "start your work," or how long it takes to respond when their name is called. This is useful when you want faster responding or better compliance with instructions. On the exam, if you see "time from instruction to response," that's a strong hint that latency is the target measure.

3.4 Interval Recording and Momentary Time Sampling

SOME BEHAVIORS ARE too frequent, too continuous, or too difficult to tally individually. Interval recording and momentary time sampling break observation time into smaller segments and record behavior in a simpler yes/no way. These systems show up a lot in RBT practice and on the exam.

- Whole-interval recording
- Partial-interval recording
- Momentary time sampling

Whole-interval recording marks "yes" only if the behavior occurs for the entire interval. For example, with 10-second intervals, you might record "on-task" only if the learner is on-task for the full 10 seconds. Any break in behavior makes that interval a "no." This tends to underestimate how often behavior occurs because partial occurrences get counted as non-occurrences. On exam questions, whole-interval is often used when you want to increase behaviors like sustained attention.

Partial-interval recording marks "yes" if the behavior happens at any time during the interval, even once. In 10-second intervals, a single second of self-injury would make that interval a "yes." This tends to overestimate behavior because brief occurrences fill the whole interval category. The exam often ties partial-interval recording to frequent behaviors that you're trying to reduce, such as repetitive vocalizations or frequent disruptions.

Momentary time sampling checks whether behavior is happening at a specific instant—usually at the end of each interval. You don't watch continuously; instead, you look up at the end of every 30 seconds or minute and record whether the behavior is occurring right then. This method is practical in busy settings because it demands less constant attention. On test items, descriptions like "observer looks at the client at the end of each interval and records if the behavior is occurring" almost always indicate momentary time sampling.

3.5 Permanent Product: Measuring Outcomes Instead of Live Behavior

PERMANENT PRODUCT MEASUREMENT uses the results or "products" of behavior instead of watching behavior in real time. This is helpful when behavior leaves a clear trace and direct observation would be inefficient. As an RBT, you may be asked to count or evaluate these products.

- Use when the behavior leaves a lasting, countable result
- Useful when you don't need to see the behavior live
- Only valid if the product clearly comes from the client's behavior

Use when the behavior leaves a lasting, countable result such as completed worksheets, cleaned areas, or items sorted into bins. For example, you can count how many math problems were answered correctly or how many chores were finished without watching the entire work period. The permanent product is the completed work itself. On exam questions, when measurement focuses on "things the client finished" rather than continuous observation, a permanent product is usually the right choice.

Useful when you don't need to see the behavior live because the outcome tells you everything you need to know. If the goal is "number of shirts folded correctly," you can inspect the stack afterward. This frees you from having to stand and watch every moment, which can be more efficient in some programs. Test items might ask which method lets you measure behavior even if you aren't present during the performance; that's a clear hint toward a permanent product.

Only valid if the product clearly comes from the client's behavior because the measure becomes meaningless if others could have contributed. If siblings, parents, or staff might complete the work, you can't be sure the product represents the client's efforts. In those cases, permanent products would give misleading data. On the exam, the correct use of permanent products usually emphasizes that the product can be attributed directly to the learner.

3.6 Preference Assessments: Finding What's Motivating

PREFERENCE ASSESSMENTS help identify what items or activities a client currently likes. While they don't guarantee something will function as a reinforcer, they give a strong starting point. RBTs often conduct preference assessments under supervision and use the results in teaching and behavior plans.

- Informal (free operant) preference checks
- Structured preference assessments (single- or paired-choice)
- Using preferences to guide potential reinforcers

Informal (free operant) preference checks let the client move freely among available items or activities while you observe what they choose and how long they engage. For example, you might put several toys in a play area and see which ones the child naturally goes to and stays with. This gives a quick snapshot of what currently interests them. On exam questions, watching what the client naturally chooses without restricting access is often described as a free-operant preference assessment.

Structured preference assessments (single- or paired-choice) systematically present items and record selections. In a single-stimulus (single-choice) assessment, you present one item at a time and note whether the client approaches or rejects it. In a paired-choice assessment, you present two items at a time and record which one is chosen, repeating with many combinations. These methods create a clearer ranking of preferences. The test may describe items presented one at a time or in pairs and expect you to identify it as a formal preference assessment.

Using preferences to guide potential reinforcers means you take items that the client strongly prefers and try them as consequences for correct or desired behavior. If the item increases that behavior, it functions as a reinforcer; if not, it might just be a preferred item that doesn't change behavior much. As an RBT, you implement what the BCBA chooses based on preference results. Exam items often ask what to do when a reinforcer "stops working"—the better answer usually involves re-checking preferences or doing a new preference assessment.

3.7 ABC Data and Descriptive Assessment

ABC DATA (ANTECEDENT–BEHAVIOR–CONSEQUENCE) are a cornerstone of descriptive assessment. They help supervisors see patterns in what happens before and after behavior, which guides hypotheses about function. RBTs are frequently responsible for collecting ABC data in real settings.

- Antecedent: what happens right before the behavior
- Behavior: clear description of what the client did
- Consequence: what happens immediately after the behavior

Antecedent: what happens right before the behavior includes events like instructions, transitions, denied access to items, or changes in environment. For example, an antecedent might be "teacher asked client to start writing," "preferred toy was removed," or "peers began a noisy activity." Recording these events helps identify triggers or conditions under which behavior is more likely. On exam questions, antecedents are the setup conditions you note before the behavior occurs.

Behavior: clear description of what the client did should be written in operational, observable terms, not as a label. You might note "client threw pencil across room and shouted 'no'" instead of "client had a meltdown." This clarity makes it easier for supervisors to understand what happened and to match it with possible functions. Test items will expect you to recognize that "behavior" in ABC data is the actual action, not an interpretation like "being disrespectful."

Consequence: what happens immediately after the behavior includes any reaction from staff, peers, or the environment. Examples include "teacher removed the worksheet," "parent gave iPad," or "staff turned away and did not respond." These consequences may accidentally reinforce problem behavior or help maintain it. On the exam, ABC questions often ask you to identify what part of a scenario is the antecedent, the behavior, or the consequence, or to choose the best ABC description.

3.8 Skill Assessment and Probes Before Teaching

BEFORE TEACHING A NEW skill, supervisors often need to know what the client can already do. RBTs may be asked to run probes or brief assessments to check baseline performance. These are not full diagnostic evaluations but simple checks of current skill levels.

- Baseline probes for specific skills
- Curriculum or structured skill assessments (under supervision)

- Using assessment results to guide starting points

Baseline probes for specific skills involve presenting a task or instruction without teaching or prompting (other than what the plan allows) to see whether the client can already do it. For example, you might say "touch red" several times with different items and record how often the learner responds correctly on their own. This gives a starting level before intervention begins. On exam questions, probes are often described as brief, pre-teaching checks of performance.

Curriculum or structured skill assessments (under supervision) use organized sets of tasks, such as language milestones, self-help checklists, or academic skills, to map out strengths and deficits. As an RBT, you might present items, record responses, and follow the supervisor's instructions, but you do not interpret scores or design the assessment yourself. Your role is to run the procedures as trained and collect accurate data. The test may ask what your role is in such assessments: implementing and recording, not designing or diagnosing.

Using assessment results to guide starting points happens when the BCBA decides where to begin teaching based on what the client can and cannot do. If the baseline shows the learner can already do the first five steps of a chain, they may start teaching at step six instead. You don't choose the starting point, but you do carry out the teaching where the plan says to start. Exam items might describe a situation where data show mastery at an easier level and ask what the supervisor is likely to do next.

3.9 Indirect vs Direct Assessment

ASSESSMENT INFORMATION can come from observing the client directly or from talking to people who know them well. RBTs should understand the difference between indirect and direct assessment and know that both can be useful. The exam may ask you to identify which type is being used in a scenario.

- Indirect assessment (interviews, rating scales, questionnaires)
- Direct assessment (observing and recording behavior in real time)
- RBT responsibilities in each type

Indirect assessment (interviews, rating scales, questionnaires) involves asking caregivers, teachers, or sometimes the client about behavior, skills, and history. Tools might include checklists, functional assessment interviews, or rating forms. These methods are quick and can provide valuable context and hypotheses but are based on memory and perception, not direct observation. On the exam, any method that relies on someone's report rather than direct observation is an indirect assessment.

Direct assessment (observing and recording behavior in real time) includes methods like ABC recording, frequency counts during sessions, and direct skill probes. These data come from watching behavior as it happens, which makes them more objective than memory-based reports. They may take more time and planning but often form the backbone of functional and treatment decisions. Test questions that show an RBT watching and recording behavior are describing direct assessment.

RBT responsibilities in each type usually involve collecting direct data and sometimes assisting with indirect tools. You may hand out questionnaires, help caregivers understand questions, or sit in on interviews, but you do not interpret results or make diagnostic decisions. Your main job is to implement direct assessment procedures as written and report what you observe. The exam often emphasizes that assessment design and interpretation belong to the BCBA, while RBTs focus on accurate implementation and data collection.

3.10 How the Exam Tests Measurement and Assessment

THE RBT EXAM USES MEASUREMENT and assessment questions to see if you can choose appropriate methods and recognize good data and assessment practices. Many items are short scenarios that describe behavior, settings, and goals, then ask what you should do or which method fits best.

- Matching behaviors and situations to the right measurement method
- Recognizing good operational definitions and ABC data
- Knowing your role in preference assessments and other assessments

Matching behaviors and situations to the right measurement method requires you to think about what is most practical and accurate. Behaviors with clear start/stop points often fit frequency or duration; frequent, continuous behaviors suggest interval recording; product-based outcomes suggest permanent product. The exam will often give several methods that could work but expects you to pick the one that is clearly best for that scenario. Pattern recognition here is a big advantage.

Recognizing good operational definitions and ABC data means you can spot objective, observable descriptions and distinguish them from opinions. Questions may ask which definition is best or which ABC recording example is correct. The strongest answers describe what happened in concrete terms without labeling the client's personality or motives. When in doubt on the exam, choose the statement that sounds most like a neutral, behavioral description.

Knowing your role in preference assessments and other assessments is crucial for ethics and scope. You are expected to help run preference assessments, ABC data collection, skill probes, and perhaps structured assessments, but not to design them or interpret them independently. The exam often places RBTs in situations where someone asks them to make a diagnostic decision or change assessment procedures. The correct answer usually involves implementing as trained and referring higher-level decisions to the supervisor.

Practice Questions – Chapter 3 (Measurement and Assessment)

CHOOSE THE **best** answer for each question.

1. Which is the **best** operational definition of "standing up without permission" in class?
   A. "Being defiant during class"
   B. "Trying to bother the teacher"
   C. "Leaving the chair so that both feet are on the floor and the student is no longer in contact with the seat during instructional time, without teacher permission"
   D. "Not liking to sit still"
2. A supervisor wants to know how many times a client shouts out during a 20-minute lesson. What is the most appropriate measurement procedure?
   A. Duration recording
   B. Frequency (or rate) recording
   C. Whole-interval recording
   D. Permanent product
3. A plan states: "Record how long each tantrum lasts from the first scream until the client is sitting calmly." Which measurement is being used?
   A. Frequency
   B. Duration
   C. Latency
   D. Momentary time sampling

4. You are asked to measure how long it takes a client to begin a task after you say, "Start your work." What should you measure?
   A. Duration
   B. Rate
   C. Latency
   D. Interval
5. A behavior happens very frequently and is hard to count each time. The BCBA instructs you to divide the session into 10-second intervals and mark "yes" if the behavior happens at any point in the interval. What type of recording is this?
   A. Whole-interval recording
   B. Partial-interval recording
   C. Momentary time sampling
   D. Permanent product
6. In whole-interval recording, an interval is scored as an occurrence if:
   A. The behavior occurs at any time during the interval
   B. The behavior occurs at the end of the interval only
   C. The behavior occurs for the entire interval
   D. The behavior occurs at least five times
7. A teacher wants to know if a student is on-task at the **exact end** of each 30-second interval. You look up only at the end of each interval and record whether the student is on-task at that moment. What procedure are you using?
   A. Whole-interval recording
   B. Partial-interval recording
   C. Momentary time sampling
   D. Duration recording
8. Which situation is **most appropriate** for permanent product measurement?
   A. Counting how many times a client swears during recess
   B. Measuring how long a tantrum lasts
   C. Counting the number of correct math problems completed on a worksheet
   D. Checking if the client is on-task at the end of each minute
9. Which of the following notes is the most **objective** description of behavior?
   A. "Client was being bad."
   B. "The client definitely hates the program."
   C. "Client hit staff on the arm with an open hand 3 times during a 10-minute work period."
   D. "The client was very rude and annoying."
10. Which of the following best describes the "C" in ABC data?
    A. The client's diagnosis
    B. The consequence that follows the behavior
    C. The caregiver's opinion of the behavior
    D. The setting where behavior occurs
11. A BCBA asks you to observe free play with several toys available and record which toys the client chooses and how long they play with each. What kind of assessment are you doing?
    A. Free-operant preference assessment
    B. Paired-choice preference assessment

C. Functional analysis
D. Interval recording

12. In a paired-choice preference assessment, your main task as an RBT is to:
A. Ask parents which items they think the child likes
B. Present two items at a time and record which item the client chooses
C. Give the client all items at once and see what happens
D. Decide which item should be the reinforcer without collecting data
13. A caregiver tells you, "When I take the tablet away, he usually screams, throws things, and then I give it back." In ABC terms, removing the tablet is most likely the:
A. Antecedent
B. Behavior
C. Consequence
D. Function
14. Which is the best example of "Behavior" in ABC data?
A. "Client is angry."
B. "Client threw the puzzle pieces onto the floor and shouted 'no.'"
C. "Client hates puzzles."
D. "Client is being disrespectful."
15. Before teaching a new skill, your BCBA asks you to present the instruction "touch red" 10 times with no prompts and record how many correct responses occur. This is an example of:
A. A baseline probe
B. Extinction
C. DRO
D. A functional analysis
16. Which statement accurately describes **indirect** assessment?
A. It always involves timing behavior in real time
B. It uses interviews, rating scales, or questionnaires to gather information from people who know the client
C. It is only done by RBTs
D. It cannot be used in ABA
17. Which of the following is an example of **direct** assessment?
A. A parent fills out a questionnaire about behavior at home
B. A teacher completes a rating scale about a student's attention
C. An RBT records frequency of aggression during a 1-hour session
D. A caregiver describes behavior from last year
18. During a skill assessment, your job as an RBT is to:
A. Design new goals based on your opinion
B. Interpret the assessment results and diagnose autism
C. Implement the assessment procedures as trained and record accurate data
D. Decide which assessment the BCBA should use
19. Which situation makes permanent product data **invalid**?
A. The client completes worksheets in a quiet room
B. Multiple people might have completed the work, and you cannot tell who did it
C. The RBT counts completed items at the end of the session
D. The supervisor creates a graph from the completed work

20. A BCBA says, "This behavior has a clear start and end, and we want to know how many times it happens per hour." Which measurement is most appropriate?
    A. Duration
    B. Frequency or rate
    C. Latency
    D. Whole-interval recording
21. In an ABC scenario, which part is the **antecedent**?
    A. "Staff turned away and did not respond after the client shouted."
    B. "The client shouted, 'I'm not doing this!' and pushed the paper off the desk."
    C. "Teacher handed the client a math worksheet and said, 'Start your work.'"
    D. "Client completed all math problems independently."
22. Why might a BCBA ask you to collect ABC data over several days?
    A. To punish the client
    B. To see patterns in what happens before and after behavior
    C. To avoid writing a treatment plan
    D. To replace all direct measurement
23. A student completes 15 out of 20 problems on a worksheet. Which type of measurement are you most likely using if you just count correct problems at the end?
    A. Frequency during live observation
    B. Duration recording
    C. Permanent product
    D. Momentary time sampling
24. Which of the following is **within** the RBT's role regarding assessment?
    A. Choosing new assessment tools without supervisor input
    B. Running preference assessments and ABC recording as directed
    C. Deciding on the function of behavior independently
    D. Writing diagnostic reports
25. Why is it important for RBTs to understand both measurement and assessment basics?
    A. So they can replace the BCBA
    B. So they can interpret all data and design treatment alone
    C. So they can collect accurate data, assist with assessments, and support data-based decisions by the supervisor
    D. So they can avoid collecting data whenever possible

Answer Key – Chapter 3 (With Justifications)

1. **C** – This definition is specific, observable, and measurable; it describes exactly what "standing up without permission" looks like.
2. **B** – Counting how many times shouting occurs in a set time frame is frequency (or rate) recording.
3. **B** – Duration measures how long each tantrum lasts from start to end.
4. **C** – Latency is the time from the instruction ("Start your work") to the beginning of the response.
5. **B** – Recording a "yes" if behavior happens at any point in each interval is partial-interval recording.
6. **C** – Whole-interval requires the behavior to occur for the entire interval to be scored as an occurrence.
7. **C** – Checking at the exact end of each interval to see if behavior is occurring is momentary time sampling.

8. **C** – Counting completed math problems after the session uses the work as a permanent product.
9. **C** – This statement describes exactly what happened in observable, countable terms, making it objective.
10. **B** – In ABC data, the “C” stands for consequence, or what happens immediately after the behavior.
11. **A** – Observing what the client freely chooses and how long they engage is a free-operant preference assessment.
12. **B** – Paired-choice preference assessments involve presenting two items at a time and recording the choice.
13. **A** – Removing the tablet right before the behavior is the antecedent in this description.
14. **B** – This describes the specific actions taken by the client, which is the “Behavior” in ABC data.
15. **A** – Presenting instructions without teaching to see current ability is a baseline probe.
16. **B** – Indirect assessments gather information via interviews, rating scales, or questionnaires from informants.
17. **C** – Recording aggression frequency during a session is a direct assessment based on live observation.
18. **C** – The RBT’s role is to implement assessment procedures as trained and record data, not to design or interpret them.
19. **B** – If multiple people might have completed the work, you cannot be sure the product reflects the client’s behavior, making the data invalid.
20. **B** – A behavior with clear start/stop points where you want “how many per hour” is best measured with frequency or rate.
21. **C** – The teacher giving the worksheet and instruction is the event that occurred right before the behavior—the antecedent.
22. **B** – Collecting ABC data over time helps reveal patterns in antecedents and consequences that may maintain behavior.
23. **C** – Counting correct problems on a completed worksheet is permanent product measurement.
24. **B** – RBTs appropriately run preference assessments and ABC recording under supervision; they do not choose tools or diagnose.
25. **C** – Understanding measurement and assessment lets RBTs collect accurate data and support supervisors’ data-based treatment decisions.

Chapter 4: Skill Acquisition – Teaching New Skills the ABA Way

Skill acquisition is about teaching clients to do more things independently and effectively in their daily lives. As an RBT, you are often the person running teaching trials, giving prompts, delivering reinforcement, and collecting data on progress. This chapter shows you how those pieces fit together so you can recognize good teaching procedures on the exam and in real sessions.

When you understand skill acquisition, you can see why plans are written the way they are and how your actions help (or slow down) learning. The exam often gives short teaching scenarios and asks what the RBT should do next, which prompt to use, or how to handle reinforcement or generalization.

4.1 What Skill Acquisition Means for RBTs

SKILL ACQUISITION REFERS to teaching new behaviors or strengthening weak ones so clients can be more independent and successful. Skills can include communication, social interactions, daily living tasks, academic skills, and more. Your role is to implement the plan your supervisor designs and make sure teaching is consistent and data-based.

Key ideas about skill acquisition:

- Focus on socially significant, meaningful skills
- Use structured teaching procedures written by your supervisor
- Collect data to show whether skills are improving

Focusing on socially significant, meaningful skills means teaching behaviors that actually make life better for the client and their family. This might include dressing independently, asking for help, following instructions, or joining play with peers, rather than random tricks that don't matter. On exam questions, the better answer usually teaches something functional and useful, not just flashy or convenient for staff.

Using structured teaching procedures written by your supervisor means you follow clear instructions about how to present tasks, prompts, and reinforcement. You are not expected to design goals or methods yourself, but you are expected to understand them well enough to carry them out accurately. When the exam shows an RBT "inventing" new teaching methods without approval, that usually signals a wrong answer.

Collecting data to show whether skills are improving lets your supervisor see if the teaching plan is working. You might track percent correct, number of independent responses, level of prompting needed, or other specific measures. The data guide decisions about when to move to harder steps, fade prompts, or change procedures. On the test, options that mention using data to adjust teaching under supervision are often preferred.

4.2 Task Analysis and Breaking Skills into Steps

MANY SKILLS ARE TOO complex to teach all at once. A task analysis breaks a big skill into smaller, teachable steps arranged in a logical order. As an RBT, you follow the task analysis to teach one step at a time or small groups of steps, depending on the plan.

Task analysis basics:

- Break complex skills into small, clear steps
- Arrange steps in a logical sequence
- Teach steps systematically and record performance

Breaking complex skills into small, clear steps makes it easier for clients to learn without becoming overwhelmed. For example, "brush teeth" can be divided into steps like "pick up toothbrush," "wet toothbrush," "apply toothpaste," "brush top teeth," and so on. Clear steps also make it easier for you to see exactly where the learner is stuck. On exam items, plans that use simple, observable steps usually reflect good task analysis.

Arranging steps in a logical sequence ensures that each step leads smoothly to the next and that the final sequence matches how the skill is done in real life. Your supervisor designs this sequence, but you need to understand it so you can present steps in the correct order. If you skip or rearrange steps, the learner may get confused or learn a version of the skill that is not useful at home or in the community. Test questions often describe correct or incorrect step orders and ask what the RBT should do.

Teaching steps systematically and recording performance means you provide opportunities to practice each step and note whether it was done independently, with prompts, or not at all. The plan might call for teaching one step at a time or using chaining procedures to connect steps over time. Your data help the supervisor see when a step has been mastered and when it is time to move on. On the exam, the correct answers usually involve following the specified teaching order and documenting each step carefully.

4.3 Discrete-Trial Teaching (DTT) Basics

DISCRETE-TRIAL TEACHING (DTT) is a structured way of teaching that uses clear, repeated teaching trials. Each trial has a beginning, a middle, and an end: an instruction, the learner's response, and a consequence such as reinforcement or correction. DTT is often used for early learning skills, but the principles apply to many kinds of instruction.

Key parts of a discrete trial:

- Clear, concise instruction (SD)
- Learner response
- Consequence: reinforcement or error correction

A clear, concise instruction (SD) tells the learner exactly what to do in a simple way. Examples include "touch car," "clap hands," or "point to red." You avoid extra words or multiple directions at once, especially when a client is still learning. On exam questions, better instructions are short and direct, rather than long, vague, or confusing.

The learner response is what the client does after the SD, with or without prompts. You watch for whether the response is correct, incorrect, or absent within the expected time window. This response is what you will record in your data for that trial. In test scenarios, the description of the learner's response often determines whether reinforcement or error correction should occur.

The consequence is what you do after the response, and it can be reinforcement for a correct response or an error-correction procedure for an incorrect response. Reinforcement might be praise, tokens, or access to a preferred item, delivered quickly and matched to the plan. Error correction typically involves calmly showing or prompting the correct answer and then moving on. On the exam, correct answers follow the plan's rules for consequences instead of ignoring errors or reinforcing incorrect responses.

4.4 Natural Environment Teaching (NET) and Incidental Teaching

NATURAL ENVIRONMENT Teaching (NET) and incidental teaching use naturally occurring situations and the learner's interests to teach skills. Instead of teaching only at a table with flashcards, you use play, routines, and everyday activities as teaching opportunities. RBTs often blend NET with more structured teaching as directed by their supervisors.

NET and incidental teaching features:

- Follow the learner's motivation and interests

- Embed learning opportunities in everyday routines
- Use natural consequences and reinforcement

Following the learner's motivation and interests means you pay attention to what the client is already drawn to, such as favorite toys, activities, or topics. You then build teaching opportunities around those interests, like teaching "manding" (requesting) for a favorite toy or expanding play skills with preferred items. On exam questions, NET options usually mention using the learner's interests instead of forcing unrelated tasks.

Embedding learning opportunities in everyday routines means you treat daily events—snack time, getting dressed, going outside—as chances to practice communication, following directions, or self-help skills. Rather than waiting for a "lesson block," you seize natural moments to prompt and reinforce target behaviors. Test items that describe teaching during normal activities are often pointing toward NET or incidental teaching strategies.

Using natural consequences and reinforcement means the outcome of behavior is something that would normally happen in that situation, like receiving a requested item or getting to continue a fun game. You still follow your supervisor's plan, but you prioritize consequences that make sense to the learner at the moment. On the exam, the "natural" option—such as giving the toy when the learner appropriately asks for it—usually reflects good NET practice.

4.5 Prompting and Prompt Fading

PROMPTS ARE EXTRA CUES that help the learner perform the correct behavior. Prompt fading is the process of gradually removing those supports so the learner responds independently to the natural instruction. RBTs use prompting systems exactly as written in the plan and are careful not to create prompt dependency.

Prompting fundamentals:

- Use the type and level of prompt specified in the plan
- Fade prompts systematically over time
- Avoid unnecessary or accidental prompts

Using the type and level of prompt specified in the plan means you follow instructions about whether to use physical prompts, modeling, gestural prompts, verbal prompts, or visual supports, and at what strength. For example, a least-to-most prompting hierarchy might start with a small gesture and only add more help if needed. On exam questions, the correct answer often uses the prompt type described by the plan, not a random choice.

Fading prompts systematically over time involves gradually reducing how much help you give once the client starts responding more accurately. You might move from full physical guidance to light touch, then to a gesture, then to no prompt. This helps the learner rely on the natural instruction rather than your extra cues. Tests often reward answers where the RBT begins to fade prompts when data show consistent success, instead of keeping strong prompts forever.

Avoiding unnecessary or accidental prompts means you watch your own behavior so you don't accidentally cue the learner by pointing, looking, or repeating instructions in a way that becomes a hidden prompt. You also avoid over-prompting when the client might respond independently. On exam items, options that mention "waiting briefly before prompting" or "reducing extra cues" usually reflect good prompting practices.

4.6 Reinforcement in Teaching New Skills

REINFORCEMENT IS A key tool for increasing new skills and maintaining motivation. In skill acquisition, reinforcement is usually delivered after correct responses or appropriate attempts, according to the schedule your supervisor sets. Choosing effective reinforcers and delivering them correctly helps learners stay engaged and make progress.

Reinforcement essentials in teaching:

- Use reinforcers identified by assessment or observation
- Deliver reinforcement quickly and contingent on the target behavior
- Follow the reinforcement schedule in the plan

Using reinforcers identified by assessment or observation means you rely on what the learner actually prefers, not what you think they should like. Preference assessments, caregiver reports, and your own careful observations can all guide reinforcer selection. Reinforcers may change over time, so you stay alert to new interests and signs of boredom. On exam questions, answers that use proven preferred items are better than those that assume generic rewards will work.

Delivering reinforcement quickly and contingent on the target behavior helps the learner connect the behavior and the outcome. The shorter the delay between the correct response and the reinforcer, the clearer that connection becomes. You avoid giving the reinforcer when the behavior was incorrect or unrelated, because that can strengthen the wrong behavior. Test items often highlight timing and contingency as clues to correct reinforcement use.

Following the reinforcement schedule in the plan means you pay attention to whether reinforcement should be delivered every time (continuous reinforcement) or only some of the time (intermittent schedules like fixed ratio or variable ratio). You do not change the schedule on your own, even if you are tired or feel like making it easier. On the exam, the RBT who sticks to the planned schedule and consults the supervisor before making changes is usually acting correctly.

4.7 Shaping and Chaining

SHAPING AND CHAINING are methods for teaching more complex or difficult behaviors. Shaping involves reinforcing closer and closer approximations to a final target behavior, while chaining involves teaching a sequence of smaller steps that form a longer behavior. As an RBT, you implement these procedures as written; you do not decide on your own which approximations to reinforce.

Shaping and chaining basics:

- Shaping: reinforce successive approximations to the target behavior
- Chaining: teach step-by-step sequences (forward, backward, or total-task)
- Follow the specific shaping or chaining plan from your supervisor

Shaping means you first reinforce a simple behavior that resembles the target, then gradually require more accurate versions before delivering reinforcement. For example, you might reinforce any vocal sound, then clearer sounds, then partial words, and finally full words. The idea is to move in small steps so the learner can succeed at each stage. On exam questions, shaping options mention reinforcing approximations, not waiting for the perfect behavior from the beginning.

Chaining means teaching each component of a sequence until the whole chain is performed. In forward chaining, you teach the first step first; in backward chaining, you teach the last step first and let the learner experience the final "success" quickly; in total-task chaining, you attempt all steps in each trial with help as needed. Your supervisor decides which chaining method to use. Test items often describe a sequence (like handwashing) and ask which type of chaining is being used or should be used.

Following the specific shaping or chaining plan from your supervisor means you do not adjust the criteria or step order on your own. If a learner is struggling, you record the data and talk with your supervisor rather than skipping steps or changing what "counts" as correct. This keeps the procedure controlled and safe. On the exam, correct answers usually involve implementing the written plan and seeking supervisor guidance when progress stalls.

4.8 Discrimination, Stimulus Control, and Teaching Concepts

DISCRIMINATION TRAINING teaches learners to respond differently to different cues or stimuli. Stimulus control occurs when a behavior is more likely in the presence of a specific cue (like a certain instruction or picture) and less likely when it is absent. Teaching concepts like colors, shapes, and categories often involves discrimination training.

Discrimination and stimulus control ideas:

- Teach the learner to respond to specific cues and ignore others
- Use clear, consistent discriminative stimuli (SDs)
- Program for flexibility and avoid rote responding

Teaching the learner to respond to specific cues and ignore others means you present multiple options and reinforce only the correct response to the relevant cue. For example, "touch red" requires touching the red item, not any item, and you reinforce only that choice. Over time, the learner learns which cues "signal" that reinforcement is available for certain behaviors. On exam questions, discrimination training often appears as "teaching the learner to pick the correct item among others."

Using clear, consistent discriminative stimuli (SDs) involves keeping your instructions and materials predictable so the learner can tell what is being asked. You avoid mixing multiple cues together, like saying "touch red and tell me your name," which confuses what behavior should occur. You also avoid unintentional cues, such as always looking at or tapping the correct item. Test items often reward the answer where SDs are simple, consistent, and not paired with accidental hints.

Programming for flexibility and avoiding rote responding means you eventually vary materials, positions, and examples so the learner responds to the relevant feature, not to a fixed pattern. For instance, you teach "red" using different red objects in different locations, not just one red card always on the left. On the exam, good answers mention mixing up positions or using multiple examples to promote true understanding, rather than teaching only one rigid version of a skill.

4.9 Generalization and Maintenance

GENERALIZATION MEANS the learner can use a skill in different settings, with different people, and with different materials, not just in the original training situation. Maintenance means the learner continues to use the skill over time, even when teaching is less frequent or reinforcement becomes more natural. RBTs have an important role in promoting both.

Generalization and maintenance strategies:

- Practice skills with different people, settings, and materials
- Gradually move from contrived to natural reinforcement
- Continue to probe skills over time to ensure they are maintained

Practicing skills with different people, settings, and materials ensures the learner does not only perform the skill with one RBT at one table. You might practice greetings with multiple staff, follow instructions in different rooms, or use many examples of the same concept. On exam questions, generalization-friendly answers involve variety and real-life practice rather than keeping learning stuck in a single, narrow context.

Gradually moving from contrived to natural reinforcement means you shift from heavy, structured reinforcement (like frequent tokens or big prizes) to more typical outcomes (like social praise or access to natural activities) as the skill stabilizes. This helps the skill blend into real life without requiring constant "special" rewards. The test often favors answers that mention thinning reinforcement or transitioning to naturalistic reinforcement under supervisor guidance.

Continuing to probe skills over time to ensure they are maintained involves checking whether the learner still has the skill after formal teaching has decreased or ended. You might schedule occasional probe sessions where you present the skill and record performance without heavy prompting or extra reinforcement. If the skill has weakened, your supervisor may restart or adjust teaching. Exam items may ask what to do when a previously mastered skill seems to be fading; revisiting and updating teaching under supervision is usually correct.

4.10 How the Exam Tests Skill Acquisition

THE RBT EXAM TESTS skill acquisition through short teaching scenarios and questions about procedures. It wants to know whether you can identify appropriate prompting, reinforcement, teaching methods, and generalization strategies while staying within your role. If you recognize the patterns in this chapter, many questions will feel familiar.

Common exam patterns in skill acquisition:

- Choosing appropriate prompts and reinforcement for a teaching situation
- Identifying DTT, NET, shaping, chaining, and discrimination training
- Staying within scope and following the written teaching plan

Choosing appropriate prompts and reinforcement for a teaching situation often means picking an answer where the RBT uses the prompt hierarchy from the plan and delivers reinforcement immediately after correct responses. You will generally avoid answers where reinforcement is delayed, given for incorrect responses, or where prompting is either absent or excessive. The correct response usually respects both effectiveness and the integrity of the plan.

Identifying DTT, NET, shaping, chaining, and discrimination training requires you to notice clues in the wording. Table-based repeated trials with fixed SDs and consequences suggest DTT; teaching during play or routines suggests NET; reinforcing approximations suggests shaping; step-by-step sequences suggest chaining; and choosing correct items among several options suggests discrimination training. On the exam, recognizing these teaching "signatures" will help you pick accurate labels and actions.

Staying within scope and following the written teaching plan remains crucial even in skill-acquisition questions. The RBT should not rewrite programs, change criteria, or add new teaching procedures independently. Correct answers usually show the RBT implementing the plan, collecting data, and contacting the supervisor if progress stalls or problems appear. If two answers look similar, the one that respects the plan and role boundaries is typically the better choice.

Practice Questions – Chapter 4 (Skill Acquisition)

CHOOSE THE **best** answer for each question.

1. A behavior plan targets "putting on a coat" using a list of small steps such as "insert right arm," "insert left arm," and "pull zipper up." This list is an example of:
   A. Shaping
   B. Task analysis
   C. Discrimination training
   D. NET
2. In discrete-trial teaching, which sequence best describes the order of events?
   A. SD → Consequence → Response
   B. Response → SD → Consequence
   C. SD → Response → Consequence
   D. Consequence → SD → Response

3. A learner only says "ball" correctly when sitting at the therapy table with one specific therapist, but not at home or on the playground. This is primarily a problem with:
   A. Generalization
   B. Reinforcement
   C. Measurement
   D. Latency
4. A teaching plan says: "Use least-to-most prompting for the instruction 'put shoes on,' starting with a gesture, then a model, then partial physical." What should the RBT do first after delivering the SD?
   A. Immediately use full physical guidance
   B. Wait briefly for an independent response, then give a gestural prompt if needed
   C. Start with partial physical prompt every time
   D. Ask the parent what prompt they prefer
5. A learner is just beginning to imitate clapping. The plan says to reinforce any movement that looks closer to clapping, then gradually require more accurate claps. This is an example of:
   A. Chaining
   B. Shaping
   C. NET
   D. Momentary time sampling
6. Which scenario best illustrates Natural Environment Teaching (NET)?
   A. Practicing colors only with flashcards at a table
   B. Asking the learner to label colors during a board game they enjoy
   C. Giving a worksheet of color names to read silently
   D. Requiring color naming drills out of context
7. A BCBA creates a forward chain for toothbrushing. Which step will typically be taught first?
   A. The last step in the chain
   B. All steps at once
   C. The first step in the chain
   D. A random step each day
8. A plan says to reinforce every correct response during early teaching of a new skill. What type of reinforcement schedule is this?
   A. Intermittent reinforcement
   B. Continuous reinforcement
   C. Fixed-interval reinforcement
   D. Variable-interval reinforcement
9. Which of the following is the **best** example of a clear SD for DTT?
   A. "Okay, you know what to do now, show me"
   B. "Do the thing we practiced before"
   C. "Touch the car"
   D. "Can you, uh, show me something?"
10. A supervisor wants the learner to respond faster to instructions. Which measurement would most likely be used to track this change?
   A. Frequency
   B. Duration
   C. Latency

D. Rate

11. A child can follow a three-step direction with one therapist in the clinic but not with parents at home. What should the RBT do?
A. Change the direction at home without telling anyone
B. Tell parents the child is just "lazy" at home
C. Report the pattern to the supervisor and assist with programming for generalization
D. Stop practicing the direction in the clinic

12. A learner has mastered a handwashing chain. The BCBA now asks the RBT to check this skill once every two weeks without prompts or extra reinforcement. This is primarily a plan for:
A. Shaping
B. Discrimination
C. Maintenance
D. Latency

13. Which situation shows appropriate use of reinforcement in teaching?
A. The RBT gives praise and a token after every correct response, as written in the plan
B. The RBT waits five minutes after each correct response to provide a reinforcer
C. The RBT gives reinforcers randomly, regardless of performance
D. The RBT withholds reinforcers to "keep the learner hungry"

14. A learner responds correctly only when the RBT points at the right answer. When the RBT stops pointing, the learner often makes mistakes. This problem is most likely related to:
A. Overgeneralization
B. Prompt dependency
C. Incorrect task analysis
D. Poor IOA

15. Which of the following is the best description of discrimination training?
A. Reinforcing any behavior that occurs
B. Teaching a learner to respond differently to different cues or stimuli
C. Teaching a long chain of behaviors
D. Asking the learner to guess randomly

16. A learner is being taught to request items. During play, the RBT withholds a favorite toy briefly and waits for the learner to vocalize or sign for it, then gives the toy. This is an example of:
A. NET/incidental teaching
B. Chaining
C. Momentary time sampling
D. Whole-interval recording

17. A supervisor tells you to switch from giving a candy after every correct response to giving it after every third correct response. This new schedule is an example of:
A. Fixed-ratio reinforcement
B. Variable-interval reinforcement
C. Continuous reinforcement
D. Permanent product reinforcement

18. In a backward chain for tying shoes, which step does the learner typically complete independently first?
A. The first step of the sequence
B. The last step of the sequence

C. A random step chosen by the RBT
D. All steps at the same time

19. A learner has just mastered a new communication skill. Which action best supports **generalization**?
A. Only practicing the skill with the same RBT in the same room
B. Practicing the skill with different people and in different settings using different materials
C. Stopping all practice now that the skill is mastered
D. Changing the target skill to something unrelated

20. A plan says: "If the learner does not respond after the SD, wait 3 seconds, then provide a model prompt." What should the RBT do immediately after delivering the SD?
A. Give the model prompt right away
B. Wait 3 seconds to allow an independent response
C. Move on to another task immediately
D. Ask the learner why they are not responding

21. A learner used to independently say "hi" to peers, but recently has stopped doing so. The BCBA asks you to collect new data and run a few teaching trials again. This is mainly addressing:
A. Measurement reliability
B. Maintenance of skills
C. Task analysis
D. Interval recording

22. Which of the following is **outside** the RBT role in skill acquisition?
A. Running discrete trials and recording data
B. Implementing NET activities as written
C. Designing new skill-acquisition goals without BCBA input
D. Following a prompt-fading plan

23. A learner can identify "red" when shown one red and one blue card, but not when shown red vs. green or red vs. yellow. What is the **best** next step?
A. Stop teaching colors; the learner clearly can't learn them
B. Only use the original red vs. blue cards forever
C. Inform the supervisor and help introduce multiple color comparisons to promote broader discrimination
D. Start teaching shapes instead

24. A teaching plan calls for shaping a greeting from "looking at the person" to "saying 'hi'." Which response should be reinforced **first** according to shaping principles?
A. Saying "hi" clearly
B. Ignoring the person
C. Any movement that indicates the learner is looking toward the person
D. A full sentence like "Hello, how are you?"

25. Why is it important for RBTs to understand skill acquisition procedures, even though they do not design them?
A. So they can design independent treatment plans when needed
B. So they can implement teaching accurately, collect meaningful data, and know when to contact their supervisor about progress
C. So they can argue with their supervisor about methods
D. So they can change goals based on their personal opinions

Answer Key – Chapter 4 (With Justifications)

1. **B** – A task analysis breaks a complex skill into small, ordered steps like those listed for putting on a coat.
2. **C** – Discrete trials follow an SD (instruction), then a response, then a consequence.
3. **A** – The learner can perform the skill in one context but not others, which is a generalization problem.
4. **B** – Least-to-most prompting starts with an opportunity for independence, then the least intrusive prompt (gesture) if needed.
5. **B** – Shaping reinforces successive approximations, gradually requiring closer versions of the target behavior.
6. **B** – Using color labels during a naturally motivating board game is an example of teaching in the natural environment.
7. **C** – Forward chaining teaches the first step first, then adds later steps as earlier ones are mastered.
8. **B** – Reinforcing every correct response is continuous reinforcement.
9. **C** – "Touch the car" is a short, clear SD that tells the learner exactly what to do.
10. **C** – Latency measures the time from the instruction to the start of the response, which is needed to see if responding gets faster.
11. **C** – Reporting the pattern and supporting programmed generalization keeps the RBT within scope and helps extend the skill to home.
12. **C** – Checking the skill periodically after mastery focuses on maintenance.
13. **A** – Delivering reinforcement immediately after each correct response as written in the plan is correct use of teaching reinforcement.
14. **B** – The learner depends on the pointing prompt; when it is removed, performance drops, indicating prompt dependency.
15. **B** – Discrimination training teaches the learner to respond differently depending on which cue or stimulus is present.
16. **A** – Using the learner's motivation for a toy in play and prompting a request is a classic example of incidental teaching/NET.
17. **A** – Reinforcing after every third correct response is a fixed-ratio schedule (FR3).
18. **B** – In backward chaining, the learner completes the last step independently first while earlier steps are prompted.
19. **B** – Practicing the skill with different people, settings, and materials promotes generalization.
20. **B** – The plan says to wait 3 seconds before prompting, allowing a chance for independent responding.
21. **B** – The skill was previously learned but is no longer occurring, so the focus is on maintenance.
22. **C** – Designing new goals is a supervisor's job; the RBT implements and collects data.
23. **C** – Broadening color comparisons and involving the supervisor supports better discrimination and generalization of "red."
24. **C** – Shaping starts by reinforcing the simplest approximation, such as looking toward the person, and builds up toward saying "hi."
25. **B** – Understanding procedures helps RBTs implement teaching correctly, gather useful data, and know when to bring concerns to their supervisor.

Chapter 5: Behavior Reduction – Safe, Ethical Support for Problem Behavior

Behavior reduction in ABA is about **decreasing behaviors that are dangerous, disruptive, or interfere with learning** in a safe and ethical way. As an RBT, you don't design reduction plans, but you are usually the person actually implementing them moment-by-moment with the client. The way you respond to problem behavior can either strengthen it or help it decrease over time, so your consistency is critical.

This chapter focuses on how behavior reduction plans are built around **function**, how replacement behaviors and reinforcement fit in, and how to follow written procedures for antecedent strategies, consequences, and extinction. The exam often gives short crisis or problem-behavior scenarios and asks what the RBT should do next, what the function might be, or which strategy is safest and most ethical.

5.1 The Purpose of Behavior Reduction Plans

BEHAVIOR REDUCTION plans exist to **decrease problem behaviors safely** while protecting client dignity and teaching better ways to meet needs. They are not about "punishing" a client but about changing the environment and your responses to behavior. As an RBT, your job is to follow the written plan exactly and communicate what you see to your supervisor.

- Behavior reduction plans focus on safety and quality of life
- Plans are based on assessment and the function of behavior

Behavior reduction plans focus on safety and quality of life by targeting behaviors that cause harm, limit participation, or disrupt learning. These might include aggression, self-injury, severe tantrums, or property destruction. The goal is to protect the client and others while making it easier for the client to access school, home, and community activities. As an RBT, you should always remember that reducing behavior is not just about stopping something "annoying" but about making life better and safer.

Plans are based on assessment and the function of behavior, not guesses or preferences. Your supervisor uses information about antecedents and consequences to identify why the behavior is happening—what the client gets or avoids by doing it. A plan that matches the behavior's function is more likely to work and to be ethical. As the RBT, you follow that plan instead of improvising your own strategies, and you provide accurate data so your supervisor can tell whether the plan is working.

5.2 Understanding Function: Why Behavior Happens

PROBLEM BEHAVIOR DOES not happen "for no reason." It is usually serving one or more functions, such as getting attention, accessing things, escaping tasks, or producing sensory experiences. Knowing the function explains why certain responses make the behavior better or worse.

- Common behavior functions: attention, tangibles, escape, automatic (sensory)
- Function guides which strategies your supervisor chooses

Common behavior functions like attention, tangibles, escape, and automatic (sensory) describe what the behavior achieves for the client. Attention means the behavior leads to social contact, such as talking, scolding, or comforting. Tangibles mean the behavior gets items or activities, such as toys or electronics. Escape means the behavior helps the client get away from tasks or situations. Automatic (sensory) means the behavior itself produces a feeling or sensation that is reinforcing. As an RBT, you don't diagnose the function, but your data help your supervisor confirm it.

Function guides which strategies your supervisor chooses, because different functions require different responses. For example, behavior maintained by escape might be addressed with strategies that teach asking for breaks and gradually increasing tolerance for tasks, while attention-maintained behavior might be addressed by teaching appropriate ways to request attention and not reacting to problem behavior. If you respond in ways that accidentally match the problem behavior's function—like giving attention when attention is the function—you may make it stronger. The exam often tests whether you can spot when a response is likely to reinforce the function.

5.3 Replacement Behaviors: Teaching Better Ways to Get Needs Met

BEHAVIOR REDUCTION is **never just about stopping** a behavior; it must also include teaching replacement behaviors. Replacement behaviors serve the same function as the problem behavior but are safer, more appropriate, and more acceptable to others. As an RBT, you will spend a lot of time prompting and reinforcing these replacement skills.

- Replacement behaviors should serve the same function as the problem behavior
- Replacement behaviors must be easier and more effective than the problem behavior

Replacement behaviors should serve the same function as the problem behavior so that the client does not lose access to important needs. If a child screams to escape hard work, you might teach them to ask for a break instead; if they grab toys from others for tangibles, you might teach them to request a turn. When the new behavior produces the same kind of outcome, the client has a real reason to use it. On exam questions, the best answers usually include promoting a functionally equivalent replacement, not just "stopping" the old behavior.

Replacement behaviors must be easier and more effective than the problem behavior, especially at first. If asking politely takes more effort and gets ignored while screaming works instantly, the client will keep screaming. Your supervisor designs the plan so replacement responses are reinforced quickly and consistently, making them a better option for the learner. Your role is to prompt and reward the replacement behavior exactly as written, so it feels like the easier path to the client. The test often highlights this by showing mismatches between how hard the old and new behaviors are.

5.4 Antecedent Strategies: Preventing Problem Behavior

ANTECEDENT STRATEGIES aim to **reduce the chance** that problem behavior will occur in the first place. They modify the environment, instructions, or routines to make expectations clearer and more manageable. As an RBT, you must know what to set up before and during sessions according to the plan.

- Adjust tasks, demands, and environments to reduce triggers
- Use clear expectations, choices, and reinforcement to prevent escalation

Adjusting tasks, demands, and environments to reduce triggers might include breaking work into smaller chunks, providing visual schedules, or arranging the room to minimize distractions. For clients who engage in escape-maintained behavior, the plan might include giving easier tasks before harder ones or using "first-then" structures. When you follow these antecedent strategies, problem behavior may occur less often because the situation feels more predictable and doable. On the exam, answers that use prevention strategies before behavior occurs are often correct.

Using clear expectations, choices, and reinforcement to prevent escalation involves telling the client what will happen, offering some control within limits, and reinforcing cooperation early and often. For example, you might offer a choice between two tasks or two reinforcers, or show a visual of "work then break." These moves can lower frustration and increase willingness to participate. As an RBT, you are the one actually delivering these supports every day. Test questions frequently show that good antecedent strategies reduce the need for more intense reactive strategies later.

5.5 Consequence Strategies: Responding After Behavior Occurs

CONSEQUENCE STRATEGIES specify how you should respond when problem behavior and replacement behavior occur. These responses help shape future behavior by changing what happens after each type of behavior. Your consistency with consequences is critical to the success of the plan.

- Reinforce replacement and appropriate behaviors as planned
- Follow the written consequence procedures for problem behavior

Reinforcing replacement and appropriate behaviors as planned means you consistently deliver reinforcement when the client uses the new, appropriate response or engages in desired behavior. For example, if the plan says to give a short break when the client asks appropriately, you follow that rule every time you can. This makes the replacement behavior more powerful and attractive. On exam questions, answers that neglect to reinforce appropriate behavior usually reflect weak or incorrect implementation.

Following the written consequence procedures for problem behavior means you do what the plan directs after the target behavior occurs—no more and no less. This may include calmly blocking certain responses, redirecting to a task, using planned ignoring for minor attention-seeking behaviors, or following safety procedures. You avoid reacting with extra attention, bargaining, or changes that are not in the plan. On the test, correct answers generally show the RBT responding calmly and consistently according to the plan rather than improvising emotionally driven reactions.

5.6 Extinction Basics (and Why It Can Be Hard)

EXTINCTION OCCURS WHEN a behavior **no longer produces the reinforcement** that has maintained it in the past. In a behavior reduction plan, extinction usually means withholding the specific consequence that previously followed the problem behavior, while still reinforcing replacement behaviors. Extinction can be effective but often comes with challenges.

- Extinction removes the reinforcement that maintains problem behavior
- Extinction can lead to bursts, variability, and emotional reactions

Extinction removes the reinforcement that maintains problem behavior by making sure the behavior no longer "works" in the way it used to. If attention maintains a behavior, extinction might mean not giving attention to that behavior while still providing attention for appropriate behaviors. If escape maintains a behavior, extinction might mean continuing the task (with proper support) instead of letting the behavior end it, again while honoring appropriate requests for breaks. As an RBT, you must follow extinction procedures exactly as written, because inconsistent use can make behavior worse.

Extinction can lead to bursts, variability, and emotional reactions, especially at the beginning. When a client discovers that a behavior no longer works, they may briefly do it more intensely (an extinction burst), try different forms of the behavior, or show increased frustration. This does not mean the plan is failing by itself; it may be a normal phase. On exam questions, the safe and ethical response to an extinction burst is usually to continue the plan as written, ensure safety, and communicate with the supervisor—not to give in or abandon the procedure without guidance.

5.7 Differential Reinforcement: Reinforcing the "Right" Things

DIFFERENTIAL REINFORCEMENT means you **reinforce one set of behaviors and not others**. It is a common strategy in behavior reduction plans because it helps build up better behaviors while allowing problem behaviors to fade. The exact type of differential reinforcement your supervisor chooses depends on the plan's goals.

- DRA/DRI: reinforce alternative or incompatible behaviors
- DRO: reinforce the absence of the problem behavior for a time period

DRA/DRI reinforce alternative or incompatible behaviors by giving reinforcement when the client does a behavior that either serves the same function (DRA) or cannot happen at the same time as the problem behavior (DRI). For example, DRA might mean reinforcing asking for help instead of screaming, while DRI might mean reinforcing sitting in a chair instead of running around. As an RBT, you watch for the target alternative or incompatible behavior and deliver reinforcement as soon as it occurs according to the schedule. On the exam, answers that correctly identify reinforcing a specific replacement behavior often refer to DRA or DRI.

DRO reinforces the absence of the problem behavior for a time period by giving reinforcement when the problem behavior has not occurred during a specified interval. For example, if a client goes 2 minutes without hitting, they may get a token or praise. The focus is on "zero occurrences" in a period, not on a particular alternative behavior. As an RBT, you must keep track of time and whether the behavior occurred. On test questions, DRO often appears where the plan rewards periods of no problem behavior rather than a specific replacement response.

5.8 Safety, Crisis, and Emergency Procedures

SOME BEHAVIOR REDUCTION plans include safety or crisis procedures for severe behaviors like intense aggression, self-injury, or elopement. These procedures are designed to protect everyone while respecting dignity and legal/ethical rules. As an RBT, you **only** use crisis procedures you have been trained in and that appear in the plan.

- Follow trained crisis and emergency procedures exactly as written
- Prioritize safety and dignity while avoiding unnecessary escalation

Following trained crisis and emergency procedures exactly as written means you do not invent new restraint or control methods. If a plan includes specific protective holds, blocking methods, or emergency steps, you must have been trained and monitored by your organization before using them. If you are not trained, you must tell your supervisor and not attempt the procedure. On the exam, the ethical answer is usually the one where the RBT acknowledges training limits and follows only approved methods.

Prioritizing safety and dignity while avoiding unnecessary escalation means you focus on de-escalation, prevention, and calm responses whenever possible. You avoid yelling, arguing, or using physical contact in ways that are not in the plan. You also try to protect the client's privacy and avoid drawing extra attention during crisis events. After any serious incident, you document what happened and inform your supervisor promptly. The test often rewards answers where safety, clear reporting, and respect are combined.

5.9 Documentation, Communication, and Treatment Integrity

BEHAVIOR REDUCTION plans are only as good as their **implementation and documentation**. You must record what actually happened in sessions so your supervisor can evaluate the plan. Treatment integrity (fidelity) describes how closely your actions match the written procedures.

- Document problem and replacement behaviors objectively and consistently
- Communicate concerns and implementation issues to your supervisor

Documenting problem and replacement behaviors objectively and consistently means you record what you see in clear, measurable terms, not emotional labels. You might count how many times a behavior happened, how long it lasted, or how often replacement behaviors occurred, depending on the plan. You also note significant events, such as injuries or unusual triggers, without guessing about motives. On exam questions, the correct choice usually emphasizes objective notes and data rather than opinions.

Communicating concerns and implementation issues to your supervisor includes telling them if parts of the plan are hard to follow, if you see new patterns in behavior, or if you think safety is at risk. You do not secretly skip steps or change procedures; you share the challenges so the BCBA can adjust the plan or provide additional training. Treatment integrity is improved when you are honest about what is realistically happening. The test often favors answers where the RBT reports problems instead of hiding them.

5.10 Ethics and Scope in Behavior Reduction

BEHAVIOR REDUCTION can involve sensitive, high-stakes decisions. That makes it especially important to respect your scope of practice and the Ethics Code. The exam will frequently test whether you recognize actions that are outside the RBT role or that could harm client rights.

- Stay within your role: implement, don't design or change plans
- Protect client rights, dignity, and safety in all procedures

Staying within your role means you follow the behavior reduction plan written by your supervisor and do not create new procedures, increase intensity, or add punishers on your own. If parents or teachers pressure you to "do more" or "try something harsher," you politely explain your limitations and involve your supervisor. As an RBT, you contribute by implementing, collecting data, and reporting, not by making independent treatment decisions. Exam items often highlight RBTs who overstep and ask you to choose the response that respects scope.

Protecting client rights, dignity, and safety in all procedures means you refuse to participate in any action that is clearly abusive, degrading, or outside approved methods, even if someone else suggests it. You make reasonable efforts to avoid unnecessary restraint, embarrassment, or isolation. You also follow laws and organizational policies about reporting injuries or suspected abuse. On the test, the correct answer will almost always be the one that safeguards the client's welfare and uses supervision appropriately.

Practice Questions – Chapter 5 (Behavior Reduction)

CHOOSE THE **best** answer for each question.

1. The main purpose of a behavior reduction plan is to:
   A. Punish the client for misbehavior
   B. Decrease problem behaviors in a safe and ethical way while improving quality of life
   C. Make sessions easier for staff
   D. Eliminate all challenging behaviors immediately
2. A learner repeatedly screams when given a difficult worksheet and the staff quickly remove the work. Screaming most likely serves which function?
   A. Attention
   B. Tangibles
   C. Escape
   D. Automatic (sensory)
3. Which of the following is the **best** example of a functionally equivalent replacement behavior for escape-maintained tantrums during tasks?
   A. Teaching the learner to high-five peers
   B. Teaching the learner to ask for a break using a card or words
   C. Teaching the learner to clap hands
   D. Teaching the learner to count to 10 silently
4. An antecedent strategy is best described as:
   A. A consequence given after behavior

B. A plan for what to do when behavior becomes dangerous
C. A change to the environment or routine to reduce the likelihood of problem behavior
D. A punishment that happens at the end of the day

5. A plan says to break tasks into smaller pieces and use a "first work, then break" visual. These strategies are primarily:
A. Consequence strategies
B. Antecedent strategies
C. Extinction procedures
D. Punishment procedures
6. A behavior plan states that when a learner hits to get attention, staff should **not** comment or look at the learner following the hit, but should give attention to appropriate requests. This is most likely an example of:
A. Punishment only
B. Extinction combined with reinforcement of replacement behavior
C. DRO without any replacement behaviors
D. Fixed-interval reinforcement
7. When implementing extinction, an RBT should expect that:
A. The behavior will stop immediately with no side effects
B. The behavior may temporarily increase or change in form before decreasing
C. The behavior will become less intense right away
D. Extinction has no effect on behavior
8. A plan uses DRA for aggression. Which action best fits DRA?
A. Reinforce any behavior except aggression
B. Reinforce a specific alternative behavior, such as asking for a break instead of hitting
C. Reinforce only the absence of aggression for a fixed time period
D. Punish all aggressive responses
9. A plan uses DRO for property destruction. What should the RBT do?
A. Provide reinforcement whenever any behavior occurs
B. Provide reinforcement if **no** property destruction occurs during the set interval
C. Provide reinforcement only after property destruction
D. Provide reinforcement only when property destruction is highest
10. Which of the following is the **best** example of an antecedent strategy for behavior reduction?
A. Ignoring all behavior during the session
B. Providing a clear visual schedule before starting transitions
C. Giving a time-out after every problem behavior
D. Taking away all reinforcers at the end of the day
11. A learner has been taught to ask for help instead of throwing materials. What should the RBT do whenever the learner appropriately asks for help, according to the plan?
A. Ignore the request so the learner becomes more independent
B. Provide the help or support promptly and praise the appropriate request
C. Only help if the learner looks extremely upset
D. Ask the learner to stop asking so many questions
12. A parent asks you to "spank the child if they hit you," even though the behavior plan does not include any physical punishment. What is the most appropriate response?
A. Agree in secret so the behavior stops

B. Explain that you must follow the written plan and that physical punishment is not part of your role, then inform your supervisor
C. Spank only lightly so it is not serious
D. Ask another staff member to do it instead

13. A plan says to use a specific approved protective hold if the learner attempts severe self-injury. You have **never** received training in this procedure. What should you do?
A. Try it anyway based on the written description
B. Ask another untrained staff to help you use it
C. Tell your supervisor you have not been trained and follow other safety steps you are trained to use
D. Develop your own hold that seems safer

14. Which of the following statements about RBT scope in behavior reduction is most accurate?
A. RBTs can design new behavior reduction procedures if they feel confident
B. RBTs implement written plans and collect data; they do not design or significantly change plans
C. RBTs can decide to add punishment whenever behavior gets worse
D. RBTs can independently diagnose the function of behavior

15. An RBT consistently gives extra attention and conversation to a client **after** they yell, even though the plan says to minimize attention to yelling. What is the likely effect?
A. Yelling may increase because it is being reinforced by attention
B. Yelling will immediately stop
C. Yelling will not be affected
D. Yelling will turn into aggression automatically

16. A behavior reduction plan includes blocking head-hitting and then immediately prompting a communication card that says "break please." This combination is best described as:
A. Punishment and ignoring replacement behavior
B. Crisis management without teaching
C. Safety plus teaching a replacement behavior
D. Extinction only

17. Which of the following is an **objective** way to document problem behavior?
A. "The client was awful and out of control today."
B. "The client clearly hates therapy."
C. "The client hit a staff member with an open hand 6 times during a 10-minute work period."
D. "The client is manipulative and angry."

18. A learner's self-injury suddenly becomes much more intense and frequent than usual. What should the RBT do first?
A. Ignore it and hope it returns to normal
B. Immediately design a new plan without the BCBA
C. Ensure safety, collect accurate data, and promptly inform the supervisor
D. Ask the family to stop services

19. Which example best represents differential reinforcement of incompatible behavior (DRI) for running away from the table?
A. Reinforcing any behavior that is not running away
B. Reinforcing sitting in the chair with feet on the floor
C. Reinforcing talking about feelings
D. Reinforcing hand-raising

20. A plan states: "If the learner goes 5 minutes without hitting, give them a token." This is an example of:
    A. DRA
    B. DRO
    C. DRI
    D. Extinction only
21. An RBT notices that the classroom is very noisy right before problem behavior usually starts. Which action best reflects an antecedent modification?
    A. Turning on more noise to "get it over with"
    B. Moving the learner to a quieter area or providing noise-reducing supports, as written in the plan
    C. Waiting until the problem behavior occurs, then using time-out
    D. Ignoring the environment and focusing only on consequences
22. A BCBA asks you to track how often the behavior reduction procedures are followed correctly each day. This is primarily measuring:
    A. Treatment integrity (fidelity)
    B. Interobserver agreement
    C. Latency
    D. Generalization
23. A parent insists that you "just do whatever works," even if it is not in the plan. What is the most appropriate response?
    A. Agree and experiment with new methods without telling anyone
    B. Explain your role, say you must follow the plan, and offer to have the BCBA discuss any changes with them
    C. Ask the parent to write their own plan for you
    D. Stop services immediately
24. Which situation is most likely to promote long-term generalization of a new, appropriate requesting behavior?
    A. Only practicing requests in one room with one RBT
    B. Practicing requests with different people, in different settings, and for different items
    C. Stopping practice once the behavior appears once
    D. Practicing requests only with highly unusual items
25. Why is it important for RBTs to understand the function and procedures of a behavior reduction plan?
    A. So they can change the plan based on personal opinion
    B. So they can implement it correctly, avoid accidentally reinforcing problem behavior, and know when to contact their supervisor
    C. So they can remove the supervisor from the case
    D. So they can choose any punishment they like

Answer Key – Chapter 5 (With Justifications)

1. **B** – Behavior reduction plans are designed to decrease problem behavior safely and ethically while improving quality of life, not to punish or instantly eliminate all behavior.
2. **C** – Screaming leads to removal of the worksheet, allowing the learner to escape demands, so escape is the most likely function.
3. **B** – Asking for a break directly replaces escape-motivated tantrums by serving the same function in a safer, appropriate way.

4. **C** – Antecedent strategies involve changing the environment or routine before behavior occurs to reduce problem behavior.
5. **B** – Breaking tasks into smaller parts and using "first-then" visuals are classic antecedent strategies that make demands more manageable.
6. **B** – Withholding attention after hitting while giving attention for appropriate behavior is extinction for attention-maintained behavior combined with reinforcement of a replacement.
7. **B** – Extinction often produces an initial increase in behavior intensity or frequency (an extinction burst) before improvement.
8. **B** – DRA reinforces a specific alternative behavior, such as asking for a break instead of aggressing.
9. **B** – DRO delivers reinforcement when the problem behavior does not occur during a specified interval.
10. **B** – Providing a visual schedule before transitions is an antecedent action that may prevent confusion and problem behavior.
11. **B** – Promptly providing help and praise when the learner requests appropriately strengthens the replacement behavior.
12. **B** – Physical punishment outside the plan is not allowed; the RBT must follow the plan, decline the request, and inform the supervisor.
13. **C** – The RBT must not use crisis procedures without training; they should notify the supervisor and use only trained, approved safety measures.
14. **B** – RBTs implement and collect data on plans designed by supervisors; they do not independently design or significantly change behavior reduction plans.
15. **A** – Providing attention after yelling likely reinforces it, making yelling more frequent over time.
16. **C** – Blocking head-hitting protects safety, and prompting communication teaches a safer replacement behavior.
17. **C** – "Hit staff with an open hand 6 times in 10 minutes" is a clear, observable, and measurable description of behavior.
18. **C** – The RBT must ensure safety, collect accurate data, and contact the supervisor promptly about serious changes.
19. **B** – Sitting in the chair with feet on the floor cannot happen at the same time as running away, making it an incompatible behavior.
20. **B** – Reinforcing after a set period with no hitting is DRO, which reinforces the absence of the problem behavior.
21. **B** – Reducing noise or moving the learner to a quieter space, if in the plan, is an antecedent modification that may prevent behavior.
22. **A** – Tracking how often procedures are followed correctly measures treatment integrity or fidelity.
23. **B** – The RBT must stay within the plan and role, and should direct the parent to the BCBA for any changes.
24. **B** – Practicing requests with different people, settings, and items supports generalization of the new behavior.
25. **B** – Understanding function and procedures helps the RBT implement correctly, avoid accidental reinforcement, and know when to involve the supervisor.

Chapter 6: Documentation, Reporting, and Communication

Documentation and reporting are a huge part of the RBT role, even though they can feel less exciting than direct teaching or play. Good notes, accurate data, and clear communication let your supervisor make safe, effective decisions. The exam often tests whether you know what to write down, who to tell, and how to stay objective and professional in your documentation.

6.1 Why Documentation Matters for RBTs

DOCUMENTATION IS HOW you show what actually happened in your sessions. It creates a written record that supports treatment decisions, insurance and funding requirements, and protects both you and the client if questions come up later. As an RBT, you don't decide what gets documented at a high level, but you are usually the person doing the writing.

Why documentation is important:

- Supports data-based treatment decisions
- Provides legal and ethical protection
- Keeps the whole team informed about what is happening

Supporting data-based treatment decisions means your supervisor can look at your notes and data to see patterns and trends over time. Instead of relying on memory or impressions, they can review what you actually recorded about behaviors, skills, and events. Clear documentation makes it easier to tell if a plan is working or needs adjustment. When the exam asks why documentation is required, answers that mention guiding treatment safely and effectively are usually correct.

Providing legal and ethical protection means that if there is ever a complaint, audit, or question about services, the record can show what was done and why. Good notes can demonstrate that you followed the plan, used approved procedures, and responded to incidents appropriately. Poor or missing notes can make it look like care was careless or inconsistent, even if you did the right things. On test questions, options that emphasize accurate records for accountability and client rights usually reflect ethical practice.

Keeping the whole team informed about what is happening allows supervisors, other RBTs, and related professionals to understand how sessions are going without being present every time. Your notes can explain changes in behavior, family updates, or unusual events that might affect treatment. When multiple staff work with the same client, consistent documentation prevents miscommunication and repeated mistakes. The exam often favors answers where the RBT documents and shares important session information instead of keeping it in their head.

6.2 Objective Session Notes

SESSION NOTES SHOULD describe what happened in a clear, factual, and neutral way. Objective notes focus on observable behavior and events, not your opinions or guesses about what someone was thinking. As an RBT, you're expected to write notes that another professional could read and understand without extra explanation.

Key features of objective notes:

- Use observable, measurable descriptions
- Avoid opinions, judgments, and guesses
- Include relevant details without unnecessary information

Using observable, measurable descriptions means you write what you saw and heard, such as "Client completed 8 of 10 tasks independently" or "Client hit staff with an open hand 3 times." You avoid vague statements like "Client was bad" or "Client behaved perfectly" because they don't tell anyone what actually occurred. Objective language helps supervisors and other readers interpret your notes accurately. On exam questions, you'll usually pick the option that uses specific, behavioral wording.

Avoiding opinions, judgments, and guesses means you don't write things like "Client hates me" or "Parents don't care." Those statements are interpretations, not facts, and can be unfair or unhelpful. Instead, you might write "Client turned away and did not respond to greeting" or "Parent arrived 20 minutes late for pickup without explanation." This keeps the note focused on what you can verify. The test often contrasts objective statements with emotional or biased ones and expects you to choose the neutral version.

Including relevant details without unnecessary information means you capture the pieces that matter for treatment and safety—behaviors, prompts, consequences, injuries, major changes—but skip unrelated personal gossip. For example, noting a new medication or a big change at home is relevant, but sharing your opinion about the family's finances is not. Notes should be concise enough to read easily but complete enough to tell the story of the session. On the exam, the best answer usually gives enough detail for clinical use without oversharing or wandering into irrelevant topics.

6.3 Incident and Injury Reporting

SOMETIMES THINGS HAPPEN in sessions that go beyond the usual ups and downs—injuries, severe behaviors, elopement, or serious property damage. These events usually require special incident reports in addition to regular session notes. As an RBT, you must know when and how to complete these reports according to your organization's policies.

Incident reporting essentials:

- Document what happened factually and promptly
- Follow your organization's incident report format
- Notify your supervisor and any required parties

Documenting what happened factually and promptly means you record details as soon as it is safe and practical to do so, while your memory is fresh. You include who was involved, where it happened, what led up to it, exactly what occurred, and how it was handled. You avoid blaming language and stick to observable details, like "Client fell while running; small abrasion observed on left knee." On exam questions, the correct answer usually emphasizes quick, accurate reporting after ensuring safety.

Following your organization's incident report format involves using the forms or electronic systems provided and filling them out completely. There may be specific sections for timelines, witnesses, injuries, and follow-up actions. You don't skip steps because they feel repetitive, and you don't create your own informal form instead. The test often highlights that proper reporting includes using official processes rather than casual notes or hallway conversations.

Notifying your supervisor and any required parties means you let your BCBA or designated supervisor know about serious incidents right away, not days later. For some events, your agency may also require informing caregivers, school staff, or other professionals. You follow those rules and never hide incidents to avoid "getting in trouble." On the exam, answers where the RBT documents and informs the supervisor promptly are usually correct, especially in safety situations.

6.4 Reporting Variables That May Affect the Client

SOMETIMES THINGS OUTSIDE of ABA sessions can significantly affect a client's behavior or performance. These are called "variables that may affect the client," and they can include illness, medication changes, sleep issues, or big life events. RBTs are expected to notice and report these factors because they help supervisors interpret data correctly.

Common variables to report:

- Illness, injury, or major changes in health
- Medication changes or missed doses
- Significant changes in routines or environment

Illness, injury, or major changes in health can make a client more tired, irritable, or less able to participate. If a caregiver says the child is sick, just had surgery, or has not eaten, that information belongs in your documentation. You don't diagnose, but you record what you are told and what you see. On exam questions, the RBT usually documents these health-related factors instead of ignoring them or guessing how they will affect behavior.

Medication changes or missed doses can also alter behavior, attention, or mood. If a caregiver mentions a new prescription, a dosage change, or that they forgot to give medication, you note it factually in your records. Your supervisor may need this information when analyzing sudden shifts in data. The exam often tests whether you recognize this type of information as important to document and pass along rather than dismissing it as "not ABA."

Significant changes in routines or environment include events like moving homes, a new sibling, a divorce, a caregiver losing a job, or changes in school placement. These can influence stress levels and behavior in ways that show up in sessions. When you learn about these changes, you record them in your notes and, when appropriate, tell your supervisor. On the test, you'll likely choose answers where the RBT documents major life changes as potential explanatory variables instead of ignoring them.

6.5 Communicating With Supervisors

YOUR SUPERVISOR RELIES on you for information about how plans are working in real time. Communication is not just one-way; you should actively share questions, concerns, and observations. Good communication helps catch problems early and keeps treatment aligned with the client's needs.

Healthy supervisor communication:

- Share data and notes regularly and honestly
- Ask for clarification when you are unsure
- Report safety concerns or ethical issues promptly

Sharing data and notes regularly and honestly means you provide the information your supervisor needs on the schedule your organization requires. You don't delay entering data for days or change numbers to look better. If you missed something or made an error, you say so plainly and correct it as directed. Exam items often show an RBT choosing between hiding mistakes and reporting them honestly; the ethical choice is always the honest one.

Asking for clarification when you are unsure shows that you understand your own limits and care about doing things correctly. If a plan is confusing, a data sheet doesn't make sense, or a situation arises that isn't covered, you reach out instead of guessing. You might email, message, or bring it up in supervision, depending on urgency. On test questions, the RBT who asks their supervisor for guidance when unsure is typically portrayed as acting within their scope.

Reporting safety concerns or ethical issues promptly means you contact your supervisor quickly if you see something dangerous, abusive, or seriously off-plan. You do not wait for the next scheduled meeting if immediate risk is involved. Your supervisor can then decide on changes, additional training, or further reporting. The exam frequently rewards answers where the RBT uses the supervision structure to address serious problems, rather than handling them alone.

6.6 Communicating With Families and Other Professionals

RBTS OFTEN INTERACT with parents, caregivers, teachers, and other professionals. While you are not the one making final clinical decisions, you are still a key communicator. You must balance being helpful and informative with staying within your role and protecting confidentiality.

Communication boundaries with others:

- Share session-related information in clear, respectful language
- Stay within your role when answering questions
- Protect confidentiality in all conversations

Sharing session-related information in clear, respectful language means you can describe how a session went, what skills were practiced, and general patterns you observe, in terms people can understand. You avoid technical jargon when it's not needed and speak about the client in a positive, dignified way. For example, you might say, "We worked on requesting today; your child asked for help independently three times." On exam questions, the RBT who uses respectful, understandable language with families and teachers is usually doing it right.

Staying within your role when answering questions means you do not give promises, diagnoses, or big treatment recommendations that belong to your supervisor. If a parent asks, "Should we change medications?" you explain that those decisions must go through medical providers and your BCBA. You can say what you observed but not what the plan "should" be. The test often includes scenarios where the RBT is pressured to give clinical advice; the correct answer is to redirect those questions to appropriate professionals.

Protecting confidentiality in all conversations means you only share information with people who are authorized and only share what they need to know. You avoid talking about one client with other clients' parents, and you never discuss a client in public places where others can hear details. Even with teachers or staff, you stick to relevant information and follow your organization's policies. On exam questions, the RBT who declines to share private details in a hallway or casual setting is usually chosen as correct.

6.7 Electronic Systems, Privacy, and Security

MANY AGENCIES USE ELECTRONIC health records, apps, or online systems for data and notes. While these tools can make your job easier, they also add responsibilities around passwords, privacy, and device use. As an RBT, you must follow your organization's technology policies carefully.

Electronic documentation expectations:

- Use only approved systems and devices
- Keep logins and passwords private
- Avoid storing client information on personal devices

Using only approved systems and devices means you enter data and notes into the platforms your employer has set up, not into random apps or personal spreadsheets. These systems are chosen because they meet legal and privacy standards. Typing session details into a personal notes app or sending them in regular email may violate policy. On the exam, correct answers usually show the RBT using official systems rather than informal or unauthorized tools.

Keeping logins and passwords private means you never share your account with coworkers, clients, or families. If another staff member needs access, they should have their own login, not use yours. If you suspect your account has been compromised, you follow your organization's steps to reset it and report the issue. Test questions often present situations where a coworker asks to "borrow" a login; you should choose the answer where the RBT politely refuses and follows security rules.

Avoiding storing client information on personal devices means you do not save session notes, photos, or identifying details on your own phone, laptop, or home computer unless the agency explicitly allows and secures this. If you use an agency device, you treat it with care and follow instructions for keeping data encrypted or locked. On exam items, the safe choice is almost always to keep client data within controlled systems and off personal devices.

6.8 Documentation of Program Changes and Instructions

SUPERVISORS SOMETIMES update behavior plans or skill-acquisition programs based on data and observations. When that happens, they will give you new instructions. Proper documentation of changes helps ensure that everyone is operating from the same version of the plan.

Handling program changes:

- Follow updated written plans and discontinue old versions
- Clarify and document new procedures before using them
- Avoid making undocumented changes on your own

Following updated written plans and discontinuing old versions means that once your BCBA issues a revised plan, you implement the new procedures and stop using outdated ones. You might label or archive old documents so you don't accidentally pull the wrong copy. In your notes, you may indicate that a new plan started on a specific date. On exam questions, the correct answer often emphasizes following the most recent written instructions.

Clarifying and documenting new procedures before using them means you ask questions if any part of the updated plan is unclear. You don't guess what a new term or step means; you get confirmation from your supervisor. Once you understand, you record that training or clarification occurred if your agency requires it. The test usually favors answers where the RBT seeks clarity before implementing new procedures.

Avoiding making undocumented changes on your own means you do not decide to "update" a plan because it seems easier or because someone asks you in the moment. Any change to how behavior is managed or how skills are taught must go through your supervisor and be documented. If you feel a change is needed, you share your observations and ideas with the BCBA instead of rewriting the plan yourself. Exam items often show that independent, undocumented changes are outside the RBT's scope.

6.9 Handoffs and Shift-to-Shift Communication

WHEN MULTIPLE STAFF work with the same client, how you "hand off" information between shifts matters a lot. Small communication gaps can lead to inconsistent responses, missed safety issues, or confusion for the client. RBTs are expected to contribute to smooth transitions between providers.

Effective handoff practices:

- Share key events and patterns from your session
- Highlight any safety or behavior concerns clearly
- Keep communication respectful and client-focused

Sharing key events and patterns from your session means you briefly tell the next staff member what went well, what was challenging, and any changes that matter for their shift. You might mention new triggers, successful strategies, or important caregiver comments. This can be done verbally, through notes, or in handoff forms, depending on your organization. On exam questions, the better option usually includes some kind of structured handoff rather than leaving the next person "blind."

Highlighting any safety or behavior concerns clearly ensures the next RBT knows what to watch for and how to respond. If a client attempted elopement for the first time, engaged in new self-injury, or had a major meltdown, that information must be shared, not buried in a long note. You might say, "There was a new incident of X; the plan says to do Y, and the supervisor has been notified." The test tends to favor answers where serious concerns are clearly communicated forward.

Keeping communication respectful and client-focused means you avoid using handoffs to complain about clients, families, or coworkers. Instead, you stick to behavior, data, and strategies, and you talk about challenges in a professional tone. This helps maintain a positive, team-based approach. On the exam, answers that keep the focus on client needs and objective information, rather than gossip or blame, are more ethical.

6.10 How the Exam Tests Documentation and Reporting

THE RBT EXAM CHECKS whether you can recognize good documentation and reporting habits, not whether you can write long notes under pressure. Most questions are short scenarios about notes, incident reports, communication, or confidentiality. If you know what "good reporting behavior" looks like, these questions become straightforward.

Common exam patterns:

- Choosing objective, factual documentation over opinions
- Reporting critical information to supervisors and documenting variables
- Respecting confidentiality and role boundaries in communication

Choosing objective, factual documentation over opinions often comes down to picking a statement that describes what happened instead of how someone felt about it. You'll see answer choices that say "client was awful" next to ones that say "client engaged in X behavior Y times," and the exam expects you to choose the behavioral description. Practicing this distinction now will make those questions easy.

Reporting critical information to supervisors and documenting variables means you pick answers where the RBT shares incident details, new health information, or major life events instead of keeping them private. The exam will often give you a choice between silently continuing and notifying the supervisor; the correct answer almost always includes documentation plus supervisor contact in serious cases. Remember that supervisors cannot fix what they don't know about.

Respecting confidentiality and role boundaries in communication shows up when questions involve parents, teachers, or other staff asking for information or advice. The best answers share appropriate session-related information while keeping private details protected and redirecting out-of-scope questions to the supervisor or other qualified professionals. If you consistently choose the option that protects privacy, stays within your role, and uses the supervision structure, you'll be aligned with exam expectations.

Practice Questions – Chapter 6 (Documentation, Reporting, and Communication)

CHOOSE THE **best** answer for each question.

1. Which note is the **most objective** way to describe a client's behavior?
   A. "The client was terrible today and refused everything."
   B. "The client hates therapy and tries to annoy the staff."
   C. "The client left their seat and walked around the room 4 times during a 30-minute work period."
   D. "The client was very bad and out of control."
2. Why is documentation important for RBTs?
   A. It is mainly used to criticize staff performance

B. It provides a record that supports treatment decisions, accountability, and client safety
C. It is only needed when the client misbehaves
D. It replaces the need for supervision

3. A caregiver tells you the client started a new medication yesterday. What should you do?
   A. Ignore it because medication is not part of ABA
   B. Give advice about how to adjust the dose
   C. Document the information in your notes and inform your supervisor
   D. Tell the caregiver not to mention medications to you
4. Which of the following is **NOT** appropriate to include in an objective session note?
   A. "Client engaged in self-injury 3 times during transitions."
   B. "Client completed 5 of 7 tasks independently."
   C. "The parent reported that the client slept only 3 hours last night."
   D. "Client is manipulative and does this on purpose."
5. After a serious incident where the client hit another child and caused a small injury, what should the RBT do first (after ensuring safety)?
   A. Delete the data for that session
   B. Document the incident factually and complete any required incident report
   C. Wait a week before telling anyone
   D. Only tell other RBTs informally
6. Which statement best describes **objective** documentation?
   A. It is based on opinions and feelings about the client
   B. It includes guesses about why the client did something
   C. It focuses on observable, measurable behavior and events
   D. It is written only when behavior is severe
7. A teacher in the client's classroom asks, "Can you tell me exactly what another student in your caseload is working on?" What should you do?
   A. Share detailed information about all your clients
   B. Politely explain that you cannot share information about other clients and redirect the conversation
   C. Give only the other student's diagnosis
   D. Show them your session notes
8. A coworker asks to use your login to the electronic health record system because they forgot theirs. What is the best response?
   A. Share your login just once
   B. Share it only if they are also an RBT
   C. Refuse to share your login and tell them to contact the appropriate person to fix their access
   D. Write your password on the staff whiteboard
9. A parent asks you, "Do you think we should change my child's medication dose?" What is the **best** response?
   A. Give advice based on what worked for other clients
   B. Tell them you cannot give medical advice and suggest they discuss it with their doctor and BCBA
   C. Change the dose yourself at the next session
   D. Tell them it doesn't matter what they do
10. A supervisor implements a new behavior plan and sends an updated written version. What should the RBT do?
    A. Continue using the old plan because it is familiar

B. Skim the new plan but keep following the old instructions
C. Review the new plan carefully, ask questions if needed, and start implementing the updated procedures
D. Design their own version based on what they like from both plans

11. Which of the following would be considered a "variable that may affect the client" and should be documented?
A. The RBT had a small argument with a friend before work
B. The client's parent reports that the child has a fever and did not sleep well
C. The RBT plans to go on vacation next month
D. The clinic is buying new furniture next year
12. A client's data suddenly show a big increase in problem behavior. When you ask, the caregiver says the family recently moved to a new home. What should you do?
A. Ignore the information because it is personal
B. Document the change and inform your supervisor about the move
C. Tell the caregiver that moving was a bad decision
D. Change the goal to match the new behavior without telling anyone
13. Which example of shift-to-shift communication is most appropriate?
A. "This kid was a nightmare, good luck."
B. "Client attempted to elope once during transitions; supervisor has been notified; please follow elopement procedures in the plan."
C. "You'll see what happens; I'm not going to explain."
D. "Don't worry about the plan; just do what feels right."
14. A coworker says, "Don't write that the client hit me; I don't want to get in trouble." What should the RBT do?
A. Leave the incident out of the notes to protect the coworker
B. Change the description to "client had a rough day"
C. Document the behavior accurately and follow incident reporting procedures
D. Write that the client was fine
15. Which of the following is **within** the RBT's role when communicating with families?
A. Promising that the client will no longer have tantrums in one month
B. Explaining which goals were worked on during the session and how the client responded
C. Changing the treatment plan based on what the parent requests
D. Giving detailed advice about changes to medication
16. A parent mentions that the client did not eat breakfast and seems tired. How should the RBT respond in terms of documentation and reporting?
A. Ignore it and continue as usual
B. Document the information and, if behavior is affected, mention it to the supervisor
C. Tell the parent that food is irrelevant to behavior
D. Refuse to work with the child that day
17. An RBT is unsure how to fill out a new session note form. What should they do?
A. Guess and hope it is correct
B. Ask another RBT to complete it for them
C. Ask their supervisor or appropriate person for clarification and training
D. Stop writing notes until it feels easier
18. Which is the **best** example of protecting confidentiality when using documentation?

A. Keeping printed notes in a locked cabinet when not in use
B. Leaving notes on a table in a shared break room
C. Taking photos of notes and storing them on a personal phone
D. Emailing notes to friends to get their opinion

19. A teacher asks for an update about the client's progress on classroom goals. What is an appropriate RBT response?
A. Share relevant, session-based information and, if needed, offer to have the BCBA follow up with more detailed updates
B. Refuse to share any information
C. Give the teacher detailed information about all other clients as well
D. Promise major changes to services without talking to the BCBA

20. The BCBA asks you to start documenting how often you implement a new prompting procedure correctly. What is this measuring?
A. Generalization
B. Treatment integrity (fidelity)
C. Latency
D. Interobserver agreement

21. In which situation is it most appropriate for the RBT to contact the supervisor **immediately** rather than waiting for the next scheduled meeting?
A. The client wore a different shirt today
B. The client tried a new snack
C. The client engaged in severe aggression that required safety procedures
D. The client preferred playing with blocks instead of cars

22. A client's caregiver asks you to send session notes to their personal email address from your private email. What should you do?
A. Agree and send notes from your personal account
B. Ask for their social media handle and send notes there
C. Explain that documentation must be shared only through approved channels and refer them to your organization's process
D. Print all notes and hand them to any family member you see

23. Which note best balances being concise and including relevant information?
A. "We worked."
B. "Client completed 10 of 12 trials of the requesting program independently; one brief aggression incident occurred during transitions; parent reported client slept poorly."
C. "Client was good; nothing else to say."
D. A long, emotional letter about every minute of the session

24. A coworker says they never record minor problem behaviors because it "takes too much time." What is the best action for the RBT?
A. Start skipping those behaviors too
B. Confront the coworker aggressively in front of clients
C. Continue documenting as required and share the concern with the supervisor
D. Destroy old data so everything matches

25. Why should RBTs understand documentation and reporting expectations for their role?
A. So they can avoid writing anything down

B. So they can implement documentation requirements correctly, support ethical practice, and provide information their supervisors need
C. So they can replace their supervisors in writing reports
D. So they can share client details freely with anyone who asks

Answer Key – Chapter 6 (With Justifications)

1. **C** – This statement describes observable, countable behavior with a time frame, which makes it objective and measurable.
2. **B** – Documentation provides a clear record that supports treatment decisions, accountability, and client safety.
3. **C** – Medication changes are important variables; the RBT should document and inform the supervisor without giving medical advice.
4. **D** – Calling a client "manipulative" is a judgment, not an objective description; the other options use observable facts or caregiver reports.
5. **B** – After safety is addressed, serious incidents require prompt, factual documentation and completion of formal incident reports.
6. **C** – Objective documentation focuses on observable, measurable events rather than feelings, guesses, or opinions.
7. **B** – The RBT must protect confidentiality and cannot share information about other clients; politely redirecting is appropriate.
8. **C** – Logins and passwords must stay private; the coworker must resolve their own access through proper channels.
9. **B** – Medication decisions belong to medical professionals; the RBT can suggest involving the doctor and BCBA but cannot give medical advice.
10. **C** – The RBT must follow the updated written plan, asking for clarification as needed, rather than continuing the old version.
11. **B** – Changes in health and sleep are variables that may affect behavior and should be documented and reported.
12. **B** – A family move is a major life change that can affect behavior; documenting and informing the supervisor is appropriate.
13. **B** – This statement shares specific behavior, the response, and the fact that the supervisor knows, all in a professional tone.
14. **C** – Incidents must be documented accurately regardless of staff preferences; this supports safety and accountability.
15. **B** – Describing session activities and client responses is within the RBT role; promising outcomes or changing plans is not.
16. **B** – Poor sleep and no breakfast are relevant variables; documenting and mentioning them to the supervisor if behavior changes is appropriate.
17. **C** – When unsure, the RBT should seek clarification and training rather than guessing or avoiding notes.
18. **A** – Keeping notes locked and secure protects confidentiality; leaving them out or sharing them casually does not.
19. **A** – Sharing relevant progress information and involving the BCBA for more detail respects both collaboration and role boundaries.

20. **B** – Tracking how often procedures are implemented correctly measures treatment integrity or fidelity.
21. **C** – Severe aggression and safety events require immediate supervisor contact, not delayed reporting.
22. **C** – Documentation must be shared only through approved, secure channels; personal email and social media are not appropriate.
23. **B** – This note is concise but includes key details about programs, behavior, and a relevant variable (poor sleep).
24. **C** – The RBT should continue to document as required and bring concerns about others' practices to the supervisor instead of copying them.
25. **B** – Understanding documentation expectations helps RBTs support ethical practice and provide essential information for data-based decisions.

Chapter 7: Supervision, Feedback, and Working on a Clinical Team

RBTs never work alone; your role exists inside a supervision system and a wider team. How you use supervision, how you respond to feedback, and how you communicate with others all affect client outcomes and your own career. Many RBT exam questions in this area are really asking, "Are you staying in your lane, using supervision, and behaving like a professional teammate?"

7.1 Why Supervision Matters for RBTs

SUPERVISION IS NOT just a rule from the BACB; it's the structure that keeps services safe, effective, and ethical. Your supervisor guides treatment, monitors your performance, and helps you grow over time. Understanding why supervision exists makes it easier to see why the exam emphasizes it.

- Supervision protects client welfare and quality of services
- Supervision supports your skill development and competence
- Supervision ensures accountability and ethical practice

Supervision protects client welfare and quality of services by making sure an experienced professional is directing treatment decisions. The BCBA or other qualified supervisor reviews data, adjusts plans, and monitors how procedures are used, so clients are not left with unsupported or inconsistent interventions. Without this oversight, clients could receive ineffective or even harmful services. On exam questions, the safest choice is almost always the one where the RBT involves their supervisor when treatment questions or concerns arise.

Supervision supports your skill development and competence by giving you regular feedback, training, and chances to ask questions. Over time, you learn new procedures, refine your data collection, and improve your communication skills. This ongoing learning helps you avoid getting stuck at a basic level or repeating the same mistakes. The exam often rewards answers where the RBT treats supervision as a resource instead of something to avoid.

Supervision ensures accountability and ethical practice by creating a clear structure of responsibility. The supervisor is responsible for clinical decisions, and the RBT is responsible for implementing those decisions accurately and honestly. Regular contact and observation make it easier to spot errors, correct them, and maintain treatment integrity. When a question asks who should handle a major decision or change, the correct answer typically places that responsibility with the supervisor, not the RBT.

7.2 Roles of BCBA, BCaBA, RBT, and Others

ON A TYPICAL ABA TEAM, different credentials come with different responsibilities. Knowing who does what helps you stay in your lane and avoid taking on tasks that are beyond the RBT role. The exam loves to test whether you can distinguish between RBT responsibilities and supervisor responsibilities.

- Supervisors (BCBA/BCaBA) design and oversee treatment
- RBTs implement treatment plans and collect data
- Other professionals contribute from their own disciplines

Supervisors (BCBA/BCaBA) design and oversee treatment by conducting assessments, writing behavior and skill-acquisition plans, and making changes based on data. They decide which procedures are appropriate, train staff to use them, and monitor progress over time. When serious concerns arise—like safety issues, big changes in behavior, or ethical problems—the supervisor is the one who decides how to respond. On the exam, any answer involving designing plans, conducting formal assessments, or changing goals usually belongs to the supervisor, not the RBT.

RBTs implement treatment plans and collect data, focusing on direct work with clients. Your job is to follow the written procedures as closely as possible, record accurate data, and communicate observations to your supervisor. You do not independently select new interventions or change program criteria, even if you have ideas about what might help. Questions that show an RBT inventing a plan or altering procedures without approval are typically showing incorrect behavior.

Other professionals contribute from their own disciplines, such as teachers managing classroom instruction, speech-language pathologists working on communication, or occupational therapists addressing fine motor and sensory needs. You might coordinate with them, share relevant observations, and reinforce their goals in your sessions, as directed by your supervisor. However, you do not take over their roles or prescribe what they should do. On test items, the ethical choice respects both your scope and the scopes of other professionals.

7.3 Supervision Requirements and Contact

THE BACB SETS MINIMUM supervision requirements for RBTs, and organizations often add their own policies. You don't need to memorize every percentage for the exam, but you do need to know that ongoing, documented supervision is required. You should also understand what supervision contact typically looks like.

- RBTs must receive ongoing, documented supervision
- Some supervision must involve direct observation of your work
- You should know who your supervisor is and how to reach them

RBTs must receive ongoing, documented supervision to maintain their credential. This supervision typically involves a certain percentage of your service hours and must be spread out over time rather than clustered once in a while. Sessions may include reviewing data, discussing cases, and providing feedback. On exam questions, an RBT who "never meets their supervisor" or "does not know who supervises them" is clearly not meeting expectations.

Some supervision must involve direct observation of your work so the supervisor can see how you interact with clients and implement procedures. They may observe in person or through secure video, depending on policies. This allows them to provide specific feedback and verify that plans are being carried out correctly. When the test mentions observation of sessions, it is showing this direct supervision component in action.

You should know who your supervisor is and how to reach them because you will need to contact them about questions, concerns, and incidents. If you are unsure who your current supervisor is, that is a problem to fix quickly, not something to ignore. In exam scenarios where something serious happens, the correct answer almost always includes contacting your supervisor using the established communication method.

7.4 Getting the Most Out of Supervision

SUPERVISION IS MORE useful when you treat it as collaborative rather than something to "check off." How you prepare, what you bring to meetings, and how you participate make a difference. The exam may not ask what *you prefer*, but it will test whether you act like an engaged learner.

- Prepare data, questions, and observations before supervision meetings
- Be honest about challenges and errors
- Follow up on action items after supervision

Preparing data, questions, and observations before supervision meetings shows respect for your supervisor's time and for the process. You might review recent session notes, identify patterns in behavior, and jot down any situations where you were unsure what to do. Coming prepared helps the meeting focus on real issues instead of vague feelings that "things are weird." On the exam, answers where the RBT shows up prepared and organized usually reflect best practice.

Being honest about challenges and errors allows your supervisor to support you effectively. If you struggled with a procedure, missed some data, or didn't follow a step correctly, it is better to admit it than to hide it. Supervisors expect human mistakes and are there to help fix them; hiding problems only makes them harder to address. Test questions often reward the answer where the RBT admits an error and seeks guidance rather than falsifying or omitting information.

Following up on action items after supervision means you actually implement the suggestions and changes discussed. If you agree to try a new prompting strategy or to improve data collection, you put effort into making that happen in the next sessions. You may also send updates or ask follow-up questions if something is still unclear. On exam items, the RBT who treats feedback as "homework" to apply—not just words to nod at—is the one acting professionally.

7.5 Feedback: Receiving, Responding, and Growing

FEEDBACK IS A CENTRAL part of supervision. It can be positive, corrective, or both. The way you respond to feedback says a lot about your professionalism and commitment to growth. The RBT exam often slips feedback issues into scenarios about supervision and team interactions.

- Expect feedback as a normal part of the job
- Respond calmly and ask clarifying questions if needed
- Use feedback to change your behavior in future sessions

Expecting feedback as a normal part of the job helps you avoid taking it personally or seeing it as a punishment. Supervisors give feedback because they are responsible for client outcomes and your performance, not because they dislike you. When you know this, it becomes easier to listen openly instead of becoming defensive. Exam answers where RBTs refuse or resent feedback usually reflect unprofessional behavior.

Responding calmly and asking clarifying questions if needed shows maturity and a desire to understand. If you're unsure what your supervisor means, you can say, "Can you show me what that should look like?" or "Can we walk through that step again?" This turns feedback into something practical and concrete. On test questions, RBTs who calmly engage with feedback and seek clarity are generally presented as positive examples.

Using feedback to change your behavior in future sessions is the real goal. You might adjust how quickly you deliver reinforcement, tighten up your data collection, or refine your prompting. Over time, your performance should improve as you apply what you've learned. The exam often implies that "good RBTs" show change over time in response to feedback, rather than repeating the same errors.

7.6 Working With a Multidisciplinary Team

CLIENTS OFTEN RECEIVE services from multiple professionals—teachers, therapists, medical providers, and more. As an RBT, you are part of this multidisciplinary team, even though your specific role is focused on implementing ABA plans. The exam checks whether you can collaborate respectfully without crossing boundaries.

- Share relevant information in a professional, jargon-free way
- Respect the roles and expertise of other professionals
- Coordinate with the team through your supervisor when needed

Sharing relevant information in a professional, jargon-free way means you can explain what you see in sessions to teachers or other therapists without overwhelming them with technical terms. You might say, "We're working on following two-step directions" instead of listing every ABA acronym. You focus on information that helps them support the client, not on showing off terminology. On exam questions, the RBT who communicates clearly and respectfully with other team members is usually doing it correctly.

Respecting the roles and expertise of other professionals means you don't tell a teacher how to run their classroom or a speech therapist how to design communication goals. Instead, you share your observations and follow your supervisor's guidance on how to support their work in your sessions. If there are disagreements between professionals, those should be handled at the supervisory level, not by the RBT taking sides. The test tends to favor answers where the RBT stays collaborative and humble.

Coordinating with the team through your supervisor when needed helps keep messages consistent and appropriate. If a teacher suggests changes that conflict with the plan, you can say that you must follow the BCBA's plan and offer to have your supervisor discuss it with them. This avoids putting you in the position of negotiating treatment on your own. On exam items, the correct answer usually routes significant disagreements or requests back to the supervisor.

7.7 Handling Disagreements and Conflicts Professionally

DISAGREEMENTS CAN HAPPEN—BETWEEN you and a parent, another staff member, or even your supervisor. What matters is how you handle them. The RBT exam often tests whether you can respond professionally instead of emotionally when conflicts arise.

- Stay calm and focus on facts and procedures
- Use supervision channels to address conflicts
- Avoid gossip, argument, or unprofessional behavior

Staying calm and focusing on facts and procedures means you respond to disagreements by referring to the plan, data, and policies instead of raising your voice or taking things personally. For example, if a parent questions a strategy, you can explain that it is part of the BCBA's plan and that you'll ask your supervisor to follow up. This keeps the conversation grounded and respectful. On exam questions, you'll typically choose answers that show calm, measured responses rather than heated reactions.

Using supervision channels to address conflicts involves bringing concerns to your BCBA instead of trying to resolve everything yourself. If you feel a coworker is not following the plan, or a teacher is pressuring you to break procedure, you document what you see and talk to your supervisor. They have the authority and responsibility to intervene or clarify expectations. Test items often reward answers where the RBT escalates professional conflicts appropriately up the chain, not sideways to other RBTs or down to clients.

Avoiding gossip, argument, or unprofessional behavior means you do not vent about coworkers or families in public spaces or with people who are not part of the solution. Complaining in hallways or on social media can damage trust and violate confidentiality. Instead, you keep discussions focused on problem-solving with the right people. On the exam, the ethical choice nearly always rejects gossip and public complaints in favor of formal communication channels.

7.8 Boundaries With Supervisors and Coworkers

PROFESSIONAL BOUNDARIES do not only apply to clients and families; they also apply to supervisors and coworkers. Keeping relationships respectful and appropriate supports a healthy work environment and protects everyone. The exam may include scenarios that test whether you recognize when a boundary is being crossed at work.

- Maintain respectful, professional relationships with supervisors
- Avoid dual relationships and favoritism with coworkers
- Use appropriate communication channels for work issues

Maintaining respectful, professional relationships with supervisors means you treat them neither as enemies nor as best friends. You can be friendly and approachable while still recognizing that they are responsible for your performance and for client outcomes. You avoid sharing overly personal information or expecting them to handle non-work issues.

Exam questions often show RBTs who either resist all directions or over-personalize the relationship; the best answers reflect balanced professionalism.

Avoiding dual relationships and favoritism with coworkers means you are cautious about situations where personal and work roles might mix in ways that affect fairness. For example, becoming roommates or romantic partners with a coworker who also evaluates your performance can create conflicts of interest. While the Ethics Code focuses most strongly on client relationships, similar principles help maintain trust inside the team. On test items, options that clearly blur professional roles among staff are usually not the best choice.

Using appropriate communication channels for work issues means you follow your organization's rules for scheduling, feedback, and raising concerns. You might use email, secure messaging, or scheduled meetings instead of texting supervisors at odd hours about non-urgent topics. When something serious happens, you use the emergency or escalation process outlined by your employer. The exam tends to favor answers where the RBT uses established channels rather than informal or boundary-crossing ones.

7.9 Professional Growth, Self-Care, and Burnout

WORKING IN BEHAVIOR analysis can be rewarding but also emotionally and physically demanding. Professionalism includes taking steps to manage your own stress so you can provide consistent, high-quality care. While the RBT exam won't ask about your personal self-care routine, it will test whether you can recognize when burnout or stress is affecting performance and what to do about it.

- Recognize signs of stress and burnout in yourself
- Use supervision and support systems when you feel overwhelmed
- Maintain consistency and reliability despite normal stressors

Recognizing signs of stress and burnout in yourself means noticing when you are feeling unusually irritable, exhausted, or detached, or when you start dreading sessions. These feelings can affect patience, accuracy, and responsiveness with clients. Being aware of them early allows you to take constructive steps instead of letting problems build. On exam questions, the RBT who acknowledges stress and seeks support is acting more professionally than one who ignores it.

Using supervision and support systems when you feel overwhelmed might include talking with your supervisor about workload, specific challenging cases, or situations that feel unsafe or confusing. You may also use employee assistance programs or other resources your organization provides. The key is that you do not handle serious stress entirely by yourself in ways that could harm your performance. Test items often reward answers where the RBT asks for help through appropriate channels when struggling.

Maintaining consistency and reliability despite normal stressors means you still arrive on time, follow plans, and complete documentation even when life is busy. Of course, everyone gets sick or has emergencies; the professional part is communicating promptly and following procedures when that happens. The exam typically favors RBTs who keep their commitments or reschedule responsibly, rather than those who frequently cancel or show up late without notice.

7.10 How the Exam Tests Supervision and Teamwork

THE RBT EXAM USES SUPERVISION and teamwork questions to see whether you know when to act independently and when to involve others. Most items in this area are short scenarios where you must choose the most professional, role-consistent response. If you keep the patterns from this chapter in mind, many of those questions will feel predictable.

- Questions ask who should make decisions or changes

- Scenarios test how you respond to feedback, conflict, and requests
- Correct answers keep you in your role and use supervision appropriately

Questions ask who should make decisions or changes by describing issues like modifying behavior plans, addressing major safety concerns, or changing service hours. The distractor options often show RBTs making independent decisions that belong to the BCBA. The correct answer almost always points to involving the supervisor, particularly when something important or risky is at stake.

Scenarios test how you respond to feedback, conflict, and requests from families, teachers, or coworkers. You might be asked what to say when a parent demands a change, how to respond when a coworker suggests breaking a rule, or what to do when feedback feels uncomfortable. The best choices will show calm, respectful communication that stays within the plan and routes complex issues to the supervisor.

Correct answers keep you in your role and use supervision appropriately by emphasizing implementation, documentation, and honest communication rather than independent clinical decision-making. When two answers seem plausible, look for the one that protects client welfare, respects the Ethics Code, and uses the supervision structure rather than bypassing it. That pattern will guide you through many supervision and teamwork questions on the exam.

Practice Questions – Chapter 7 (Supervision, Feedback, and Teamwork)

CHOOSE THE **best** answer for each question.

1. Which statement best describes the RBT's relationship to supervision?
   A. Supervision is optional if the RBT is experienced
   B. Supervision is required and ensures that a qualified professional directs treatment
   C. Supervision is only needed when there are serious problems
   D. Supervision exists mainly to catch staff doing things wrong
2. Which task is **within** the RBT role?
   A. Writing a new behavior plan when problem behavior increases
   B. Changing treatment goals based on parent requests
   C. Implementing existing plans and collecting data as written
   D. Determining which assessments should be conducted
3. A parent asks you to change the behavior plan because they "don't like it" and want you to "do something different." What is the best response?
   A. Agree and change the plan yourself
   B. Explain that you must follow the BCBA's plan and offer to have your supervisor discuss changes with them
   C. Say no and refuse to talk about it
   D. Tell them to design their own plan
4. Which behavior during supervision best reflects professional use of feedback?
   A. Arguing with the supervisor about every suggestion
   B. Listening, asking clarifying questions, and making an effort to apply the feedback
   C. Nodding politely but changing nothing afterward
   D. Refusing to attend supervision meetings
5. A teacher asks you to "ignore what the BCBA said" and use a different strategy they prefer. What should you do?
   A. Follow the teacher's idea to keep them happy
   B. Combine both plans however you think is best

C. Explain that you must follow the BCBA's plan and offer to have your supervisor talk with the teacher
D. Stop running the program altogether

6. Which of the following is an appropriate way for an RBT to communicate with a teacher about progress?
   A. "We worked on following two-step directions today; your student followed 8 of 10 independently."
   B. "I can't tell you anything; it's all confidential."
   C. "Your student is terrible during therapy."
   D. "I'll change the goals tomorrow to match your preferences."
7. A coworker complains loudly about a client and family in the staff room and invites you to join in. What is the most professional action?
   A. Join the conversation and add your own complaints
   B. Laugh along but say nothing
   C. Avoid participating and, if the behavior continues, bring the concern to your supervisor
   D. Post the story on social media instead
8. You are unsure how to implement a new prompting hierarchy that was just added to the plan. What should you do?
   A. Guess and hope you are correct
   B. Ask your supervisor for clarification and training
   C. Design a different prompting system that seems easier
   D. Ignore the change and keep using the old prompts
9. A BCBA from another agency asks you for detailed information about your client's treatment without any release of information on file. What should you do?
   A. Share everything to help the client
   B. Provide only the diagnosis
   C. Explain that you cannot share information without proper authorization and refer them to your supervisor
   D. Email them your notes from your personal account
10. A supervisor observes your session and notes that you are delivering reinforcement several minutes after correct responses. What is the best way to respond to this feedback?
    A. Say they are wrong and you will not change
    B. Ask for examples of how to deliver reinforcement more immediately and practice the new timing
    C. Quit your job
    D. Ignore the feedback and continue as before
11. In which situation should the RBT contact their supervisor **immediately** rather than waiting for the next scheduled meeting?
    A. You forgot your favorite pen at home
    B. A client tried a new snack at lunch
    C. A client engaged in severe aggression requiring emergency procedures
    D. A client chose a different reinforcer than usual
12. Which scenario best respects the roles of other professionals?
    A. Telling the speech therapist how they should write communication goals
    B. Working on ABA goals while coordinating with the speech therapist through your supervisor
    C. Ignoring what the teacher says about classroom behavior
    D. Giving the teacher instructions on how to grade assignments
13. A BCBA schedules a supervision meeting to review your data. Which behavior is **most** professional?
    A. Arrive without data and hope they don't notice

B. Cancel at the last minute without explanation
C. Arrive on time with organized data and questions about cases
D. Refuse to attend because you "already know what to do"

14. Which example best shows staying within professional boundaries with a supervisor?
    A. Expecting your supervisor to handle your personal problems
    B. Developing a romantic relationship with your supervisor
    C. Treating the supervisor respectfully, discussing work matters openly, and keeping personal topics limited
    D. Ignoring all emails from your supervisor
15. You notice a coworker regularly ignores parts of the behavior plan and uses their own methods instead. What should you do?
    A. Use their methods so everyone is consistent
    B. Yell at them in front of the client
    C. Continue following the plan yourself and report your observations to your supervisor
    D. Change the written plan to match what the coworker is doing
16. A parent asks you to be their child's regular babysitter on weekends. What is the best response?
    A. Accept so you can earn extra money
    B. Accept as long as you don't mention ABA
    C. Politely decline and explain that this would create a dual relationship and is not appropriate for your role
    D. Agree if the BCBA doesn't find out
17. Which statement about RBT scope is most accurate?
    A. RBTs can independently diagnose autism
    B. RBTs can change treatment plans without telling anyone
    C. RBTs implement plans and report data; supervisors design and change plans
    D. RBTs can take over cases if a BCBA is unavailable
18. A teacher disagrees with a strategy in the plan and becomes frustrated. What is the most appropriate RBT action?
    A. Argue until the teacher agrees
    B. Ignore the teacher's concerns completely
    C. Listen respectfully, explain that you must follow the plan, and offer to have the BCBA meet with them
    D. Immediately change the strategy to whatever the teacher wants
19. Which example best reflects using supervision to handle personal stress that is affecting your work?
    A. Hiding your stress and letting your performance decline
    B. Discussing with your supervisor that you are feeling overwhelmed and asking for guidance
    C. Venting about clients on social media
    D. Stopping data collection when you feel tired
20. A coworker invites you to share drinks after work and discuss "how annoying some families are." What is the best professional response?
    A. Go and openly complain about families
    B. Decline or redirect the conversation to neutral topics if you go, avoiding unprofessional gossip
    C. Take notes and share them with families
    D. Record the conversation and post it online
21. A scheduling change means you will be late to a session. What is the most professional way to handle it?
    A. Arrive late without telling anyone
    B. Not show up and explain later

C. Notify the appropriate person as soon as you know and follow your organization's procedures for rescheduling or adjusting times
D. Ask a friend to go in your place

22. A BCBA from your agency gives you feedback that feels hard to hear but is focused on client care. What should you do?
A. Immediately argue and say they are wrong
B. Leave the session without speaking
C. Listen, ask for clarification if needed, and try to implement the feedback
D. Tell families you disagree with the BCBA
23. During a team meeting, you disagree with a suggestion but you are the only RBT present. What is the best way to express this?
A. Shout that everyone else is wrong
B. Say nothing and complain later to coworkers
C. Calmly share your observations, then defer final decisions to the supervisor
D. Announce that you will do whatever you want in your sessions
24. A new BCBA takes over your case and updates the plan. What is your best course of action?
A. Refuse to work with the new BCBA
B. Continue to use the old plan because you liked it better
C. Review the updated plan, ask questions if needed, and follow the new procedures
D. Mix pieces from both plans based on your preferences
25. Why is it important for RBTs to understand supervision and teamwork expectations?
A. So they can replace the BCBA
B. So they can make all decisions independently
C. So they can work effectively within their role, protect client welfare, and use the support of the team appropriately
D. So they can avoid communicating with others

Answer Key – Chapter 7 (With Justifications)

1. **B** – Supervision is required and ensures that a qualified professional directs treatment while the RBT implements it.
2. **C** – Implementing existing plans and collecting data fall squarely within the RBT role; designing plans does not.
3. **B** – The RBT must follow the BCBA's plan and route requests for changes to the supervisor, not change the plan alone.
4. **B** – Listening, clarifying, and applying feedback shows professional use of supervision.
5. **C** – The RBT must follow the BCBA's plan and offer to connect the teacher with the supervisor to discuss concerns.
6. **A** – Sharing clear, factual progress information with the teacher in simple language is appropriate.
7. **C** – Avoiding gossip and, if necessary, bringing concerns to the supervisor supports professionalism and ethics.
8. **B** – When unsure, the RBT should seek training and clarification from the supervisor rather than guessing or ignoring changes.
9. **C** – The RBT must protect confidentiality and cannot release information without proper authorization; the

supervisor should handle such requests.

10. **B** – Asking for concrete guidance and practicing new timing shows constructive response to feedback.
11. **C** – Severe aggression requiring emergency procedures is a serious event that demands immediate supervisor contact.
12. **B** – Coordinating through your supervisor respects both your ABA role and the other professional's expertise.
13. **C** – Arriving prepared with data and questions demonstrates professional engagement with supervision.
14. **C** – A respectful, work-focused relationship that maintains boundaries is appropriate with a supervisor.
15. **C** – Continuing to follow the plan and reporting non-compliance to the supervisor is the ethical choice.
16. **C** – Babysitting creates a dual relationship; politely declining and citing professional boundaries is correct.
17. **C** – RBTs implement plans and report data; supervisors design and modify plans and handle higher-level clinical decisions.
18. **C** – Listening respectfully, explaining your constraints, and involving the BCBA balances collaboration with role boundaries.
19. **B** – Discussing overwhelming stress with your supervisor and asking for guidance uses support systems appropriately.
20. **B** – Avoiding unprofessional gossip, even in social settings, maintains ethical boundaries.
21. **C** – Notifying the right person and following procedures for scheduling changes is professional and respectful.
22. **C** – Listening and trying to apply feedback, even when it is difficult to hear, shows professionalism.
23. **C** – Calmly sharing observations while deferring to the supervisor for final decisions keeps you in your role.
24. **C** – Reviewing and implementing the updated plan, with questions as needed, aligns with expectations when supervision changes.
25. **C** – Understanding supervision and teamwork helps RBTs work effectively within their scope and protect client welfare using the team's support.

Chapter 8: RBT Exam Strategy, Study Plans, and Next Steps

The RBT exam isn't just about what you know; it's also about how you **prepare** and **take the test**. You've already seen the main content areas—measurement, skill acquisition, behavior reduction, documentation, ethics, and supervision. This chapter focuses on turning that content into a realistic study plan and exam strategy so you can walk into the test as calm and prepared as possible.

You'll look at how the exam is structured, how to study efficiently, how to handle scenario questions, and what to do on exam day itself. Think of this chapter as your "operations manual" for getting from where you are now to a passing score and a smooth start as an RBT.

8.1 Understanding the Exam Structure

KNOWING WHAT THE EXAM looks like helps you study in a focused way instead of guessing. When you understand that questions are multiple-choice, scenario-based, and mapped to the RBT Task List, you can tailor your practice to match that style. The goal is not to memorize trivia but to be comfortable with how questions are asked.

Big exam structure points:

- Computer-based, multiple-choice test
- Questions tied to the RBT Task List domains
- Heavy use of short, realistic scenarios

A computer-based, multiple-choice test means you'll be reading questions on a screen and selecting from fixed options rather than writing essays or doing oral responses. You won't have partial credit—each question has one best answer—so your task is to narrow down choices logically. Knowing the format lets you practice with similar question types and get used to reading carefully instead of skimming.

Questions tied to the RBT Task List domains means content is organized around the same areas you've been studying: measurement, assessment basics, skill acquisition, behavior reduction, documentation and reporting, and professional conduct/scope of practice. That doesn't mean you'll see section labels on the exam, but it does mean you can structure your study in the same way: review a domain, then do targeted practice questions. By mapping your studying to those domains, you reduce the chance of big blind spots.

Heavy use of short, realistic scenarios means many questions will look like mini stories from sessions you might have in real life. They're not just asking for definitions; they're checking if you can recognize what an ethical RBT would do. That's why this book keeps giving you "what should you do next?" questions. The more you practice seeing patterns in these scenarios, the easier exam questions will feel.

8.2 Building a Realistic Study Plan

A GOOD STUDY PLAN HELPS you cover everything without burning out or cramming at the last minute. You don't need a perfect, fancy plan; you need something you can actually follow. The best plans break the content into pieces, schedule practice, and build in review.

Effective study plan elements:

- Set a realistic timeline with regular, shorter study sessions
- Rotate through content domains instead of cramming one area
- Include practice questions and self-checks in each study block

Setting a realistic timeline with regular, shorter study sessions means choosing a period (for example, 3–6 weeks) and planning several 30–60 minute blocks each week. Marathon sessions once in a while are less effective than steady, repeated exposure to the material. You're aiming for consistency, not perfection. Even two focused evenings a week plus a chunk on the weekend can add up quickly.

Rotating through content domains instead of cramming one area helps your brain connect ideas and prevents boredom. One night might focus on measurement and graphs, another on skill acquisition, and another on ethics and scope. You can still go deeper into tough domains, but you don't want to ignore others for so long that they become rusty. A simple rotation keeps everything "warm" in your memory.

Including practice questions and self-checks in each study block makes your studying active instead of passive. Reading is useful, but doing questions forces you to retrieve information and apply it, which is exactly what the exam requires. After a short reading or review, you can answer a few questions, then immediately look at explanations to see why each answer is right or wrong. That feedback loop is where a lot of learning happens.

8.3 Using Practice Questions the Right Way

PRACTICE QUESTIONS can be powerful tools—or just more noise—depending on how you use them. You're not just trying to "get a high score" on practice sets; you're trying to train your brain to recognize patterns in how exam questions are written. The process matters as much as the result.

Smart practice question habits:

- Answer questions in exam-like conditions when possible
- Review explanations for both correct and incorrect answers
- Track patterns in your mistakes and adjust your studying

Answering questions in exam-like conditions when possible means sometimes doing timed sets, not checking answers until you've finished a block, and working without distractions. You don't need to simulate the full exam every time, but you want to get used to reading carefully and committing to answers without instantly peeking. This helps you manage nerves and pace yourself.

Reviewing explanations for both correct and incorrect answers helps you understand the logic of the question rather than just "getting it right by luck." Even when you choose the correct answer, reading why it is correct and why the others are wrong deepens your understanding. Over time, you'll start noticing that the exam often rewards certain patterns: respect scope, follow the plan, protect confidentiality, use data, contact your supervisor appropriately.

Tracking patterns in your mistakes and adjusting your studying turns practice questions into a personalized study guide. If you keep missing items about measurement, you know to revisit Chapter 3. If ethics questions trip you up, Chapters 2 and 5 need another pass. You can keep a quick list of "things to review" as you grade practice sets, then deliberately target those weak spots in your next study block.

8.4 Reading Questions Carefully and Avoiding Traps

MANY EXAM QUESTIONS are not hard because of the content but because of how they're worded. Small details—like "what should you do first?" or "most appropriate"—can change the answer. Learning to slow down and read the full question carefully is a big part of test success.

Question-reading strategies:

- Pay attention to key words like "first," "best," or "most ethical"
- Separate what the plan says from what others are pressuring you to do
- Eliminate obviously wrong options before choosing your answer

Paying attention to key words like "first," "best," or "most ethical" prevents you from picking an answer that might be okay but not the best choice in that situation. For example, "what should you do first?" usually favors immediate safety or clear documentation, not longer-term steps. If you ignore those words, you may choose something helpful but out of order. Underline or mentally highlight those qualifiers as you read.

Separating what the plan says from what others are pressuring you to do is a common exam theme. Many scenarios show teachers, parents, or coworkers urging you to break the plan or act outside your role. The exam wants to see if you can recognize that you must still follow the written procedures and bring concerns to your supervisor. If an option says to ignore the plan or "just try something else," that's almost always a red flag.

Eliminating obviously wrong options before choosing your answer simplifies tricky questions. Often, two choices will be clearly wrong (because they break ethics, violate scope, or ignore safety), leaving you with two more reasonable options. At that point, looking for the one that best protects client rights, uses supervision, and follows the plan will usually lead you to the correct answer. The process of elimination is a skill you can practice.

8.5 Focusing on High-Yield Content Areas

NOT EVERY TINY DETAIL is equally likely to appear on the exam. Some topics—like reinforcement, measurement, ethics, and scope of practice—tend to show up again and again in different forms. Focusing extra attention on these "high-yield" areas is a smart strategy.

High-yield content topics:

- Measurement and basic graphs
- Reinforcement, prompting, and basic teaching procedures
- Ethics, professionalism, and scope of practice

Measurement and basic graphs are core RBT skills because they tie directly to your daily work. Frequency, duration, latency, interval recording, permanent products, and reading simple trends all show up frequently. If you can choose the right measurement method and interpret a simple graph, you'll be ready for a big slice of exam questions in that domain. Don't skip over these basics thinking they're "too easy."

Reinforcement, prompting, and basic teaching procedures underpin all of skill acquisition. Questions will ask when to deliver reinforcement, how to fade prompts, and how to apply methods like DTT and NET in real scenarios. These topics connect directly to Chapters 3, 4, and 5, and they show up across many domains—sometimes even inside ethics and supervision questions. Knowing these tools well makes many questions feel familiar.

Ethics, professionalism, and scope of practice are huge because the BACB cares deeply about how services are delivered, not just what is taught. Many exam items are essentially asking, "Did the RBT act within their role and uphold the Ethics Code?" That's why there are entire chapters here on ethics, documentation, behavior reduction, and supervision. If you can consistently choose answers that protect client rights and stay in your lane, you're in good shape.

8.6 Managing Test Anxiety and Staying Focused

EVEN IF YOU KNOW THE material, anxiety can make it harder to retrieve information and think clearly. Test anxiety is common, and it doesn't mean you're unprepared; it just means you need a few strategies to manage nerves. The exam doesn't test your emotions, but managing them helps you show what you actually know.

Test-anxiety management tips:

- Practice under mild pressure so the real test feels familiar
- Use simple breathing or grounding techniques before and during the exam
- Focus on one question at a time instead of the whole test at once

Practicing under mild pressure means occasionally doing timed practice sets, maybe sitting in a quiet place with your phone away, so you get used to a more formal environment. You don't have to duplicate exam conditions perfectly; just create situations where you take practice seriously and feel a little bit of performance pressure. When exam day comes, the environment will feel less strange.

Using simple breathing or grounding techniques before and during the exam can calm your nervous system enough to think clearly. This might be as simple as inhaling slowly for a count of four, exhaling for a count of six, and repeating a few times. You can also quietly remind yourself, "I've studied this; I just need to read carefully and choose the best answer." These aren't magic, but they can keep anxiety from snowballing.

Focusing on one question at a time instead of the whole test at once helps prevent overwhelm. You don't need to know all 25 or 30 questions on a screen; you just need to do your best on this one, then move to the next. If you hit a tough question, make your best choice, mark it if the system allows, and move on rather than getting stuck. Often, later questions jog your memory and help you come back with clearer thinking.

8.7 Exam Day Logistics and Mindset

PRACTICAL DETAILS CAN make exam day smoother or more stressful than it needs to be. Knowing what to expect helps you avoid last-minute surprises and lets you focus on the questions instead of logistics. Think of this as the "operational readiness" part of your plan.

Exam day essentials:

- Know where you're going and what you need to bring
- Arrive early and give yourself time to settle
- Adopt a calm, confident mindset—even if you feel nervous inside

Knowing where you're going and what you need to bring means checking the testing center address, ID requirements, and any guidelines about personal items ahead of time. Don't wait until the morning of the exam to look up directions or find your identification. Taking care of these details early leaves you with more bandwidth for the actual test.

Arriving early and giving yourself time to settle lets you adjust to the testing environment, use the restroom, and take a few deep breaths before starting. Rushing in at the last minute tends to spike anxiety and make you feel scattered. Aim to get there with a comfortable cushion, not so early that you're sitting for hours, but enough time to decompress.

Adopting a calm, confident mindset—even if you feel nervous inside—is about how you talk to yourself. Instead of thinking, "If I miss one question, I'll fail," you can remind yourself, "I've done the work; I don't need to be perfect, just solid." Nervousness doesn't mean you're going to fail; lots of people pass while feeling anxious. The key is to manage that anxiety rather than letting it dictate your actions.

8.8 During the Exam: Pacing, Guessing, and Review

ONCE THE EXAM BEGINS, your job shifts from preparation to execution. How you use your time and handle tough questions matters. A steady pace and a clear strategy for guessing and reviewing can make a real difference.

In-exam strategies:

- Pace yourself so you don't rush or run out of time
- Make educated guesses rather than leaving questions blank
- Use review features (if available) to revisit marked questions

Pacing yourself so you don't rush or run out of time means checking how many questions you have and how much time is available, then keeping a rough mental clock. If you find yourself stuck on one question for too long, it may be better to choose the best answer you can and move on, then come back later if the system allows. Staying aware of time—without obsessing over it—helps you avoid the panic of seeing lots of unanswered questions at the end.

Making educated guesses rather than leaving questions blank is important because most multiple-choice exams don't penalize you for guessing, but they do for unanswered questions. You can use elimination to rule out clearly unethical, unsafe, or out-of-scope options, then choose from what remains. Even if you're not certain, a thoughtful guess is far better than skipping the item.

Using review features (if available) to revisit marked questions allows you to manage uncertainty without getting stuck. If you're really unsure, choose your best answer, mark the question (if there's a flagging system), and move on. Later, you might have time and a calmer head to re-read those questions and refine your answers. Just remember: changing answers is helpful only if you have a specific reason, not just vague doubt.

8.9 After the Exam: Next Steps and Continuous Growth

NO MATTER HOW THE EXAM goes, your career as an RBT is about more than one test. If you pass, you'll start or continue working in the field; if you don't pass yet, that's feedback about what to study more deeply. Either way, growth and learning continue.

Post-exam mindset:

- See the exam as one step in a longer career path
- Use results (pass or fail) as information about strengths and gaps
- Keep building skills through supervision and ongoing learning

Seeing the exam as one step in a longer career path helps keep it in perspective. Passing is important, but your day-to-day performance, ethics, and professionalism matter just as much for your clients and your reputation. Even after you're certified, you'll still be learning from supervisors, coworkers, and clients. The exam is the starting line, not the finish line.

Using results (pass or fail) as information about strengths and gaps lets you turn any outcome into something useful. If you pass, you can reflect on which domains felt easiest and which felt toughest, then focus on future learning where you felt shaky. If you don't pass yet, your score report and your own memory of the exam can guide a more targeted study plan for next time. The key is to avoid turning results into a judgment of your worth; they're just data.

Keeping building skills through supervision and ongoing learning means treating every supervision meeting, training, and case as an opportunity to deepen your understanding. Over time, concepts like function, reinforcement, ethics, and measurement will feel more natural because you've applied them many times. That continuous growth makes you more effective with clients and may open doors to future credentials if you choose to pursue them.

8.10 Putting It All Together: Content + Strategy

THE RBT EXAM TESTS **both** your knowledge and your decision-making. Passing requires understanding the core ABA concepts and being able to apply them in realistic situations under time pressure. This chapter has focused on the strategy side—how to study, how to read questions, and how to handle the test environment.

Success formula for the RBT exam:

- Solid understanding of core content domains
- Consistent, targeted practice with scenario-based questions
- Calm, strategic approach to exam day and question answering

Solid understanding of core content domains comes from working through chapters like the ones in this book, doing training, and getting supervised experience. You don't need to be a BCBA-level expert, but you do need to be comfortable with basic measurement, teaching, behavior reduction, ethics, documentation, and supervision. That content knowledge is the foundation of your exam performance and your future work.

Consistent, targeted practice with scenario-based questions turns that knowledge into exam-ready skill. By working on realistic vignettes, you get used to spotting patterns like "follow the plan," "stay in scope," "protect confidentiality," "use data," and "contact your supervisor." Over time, those patterns feel automatic, and many exam questions become easier to interpret.

Calm, strategic approach to exam day and question answering ties everything together. With a clear study plan, good test-taking habits, and a reasonable mindset, you give yourself the best chance to show what you know. Even if you feel nervous, you can use pacing, elimination, and careful reading to navigate the test. Put content, practice, and strategy together, and you're well-positioned to succeed.

Mock RBT Practice Exam A (85 Questions)

Instructions

- This mock exam is designed to mirror the **length and style** of the RBT certification exam.
- There are **85 multiple-choice questions**. Each question has **one best answer**.
- Choose the **single best answer (A, B, C, or D)** for each item.
- Some questions may have more than one answer that seems "okay" — select the answer that is **most consistent with the RBT Task List, ethics, and scope of practice.**
- You can time yourself (for pacing practice) or work untimed and focus on careful reading.
- After finishing, check the **answer key** and read the brief justifications to understand why each correct answer is best.

Questions

1. A behavior plan defines "tantrum" as "falling to the floor, crying loudly, and/or kicking the floor or furniture for at least 10 seconds." This is an example of:
   A. A diagnosis
   B. An operational definition
   C. A consequence
   D. A reinforcement schedule
2. Your supervisor wants to know how many times a client elopes (leaves the table) during a 1-hour session. Which measurement is most appropriate?
   A. Duration
   B. Frequency or rate
   C. Whole-interval recording
   D. Permanent product
3. A BCBA asks you to time how long each math work period lasts before the client leaves their seat. What type of measurement is this?
   A. Frequency
   B. Duration
   C. Latency
   D. Momentary time sampling
4. You say, "Touch your nose," and start a timer. You stop the timer when the client touches their nose. What did you measure?
   A. Frequency
   B. Latency
   C. Duration
   D. Rate
5. A client engages in hand-flapping so frequently that you cannot count every instance. The BCBA instructs you to mark "yes" if it occurs at any time during each 15-second interval. This is:
   A. Whole-interval recording
   B. Partial-interval recording

C. Momentary time sampling
D. Permanent product

6. A teacher wants to know if a student is on-task at the exact moment each 1-minute interval ends. Which method should you use?
A. Duration recording
B. Whole-interval recording
C. Partial-interval recording
D. Momentary time sampling
7. Which of the following is **most appropriate** for permanent product recording?
A. Counting how many times the client yells
B. Timing how long a tantrum lasts
C. Counting completed chores at the end of the day
D. Checking if the client is on-task during every minute
8. During play, you set out 8 different toys and let the client roam freely. You record which toys they approach and how long they use each one. What kind of assessment is this?
A. Paired-choice preference assessment
B. Free-operant preference assessment
C. Functional analysis
D. Interval recording
9. In a paired-choice preference assessment, your job as an RBT is to:
A. Ask parents which reinforcers to use
B. Present two items at a time and record which one is chosen
C. Present all items at once and count how loud the client laughs
D. Decide which items to throw away
10. The "A" in ABC data stands for:
A. Antecedent
B. After-effect
C. Attention
D. Assessment
11. A caregiver says, "He throws his cup every time I say 'no more juice,' and then I usually pour more." In ABC terms, "no more juice" is the:
A. Behavior
B. Consequence
C. Antecedent
D. Function
12. Which of the following is **direct assessment**?
A. A parent completes a behavior checklist from memory
B. A teacher fills out a rating scale about attention
C. An RBT records the number of times a client hits during a session
D. A caregiver talks about behavior from last year
13. Before starting a new program for "identifying animals," the BCBA has you present 10 animal pictures with the SD "What is this?" and record correct answers, without teaching. This is a:
A. Functional analysis
B. Baseline probe

C. DRO procedure
D. Extinction burst

14. During discrete-trial teaching, what is the correct order of events in a trial?
A. Response → Consequence → SD
B. SD → Response → Consequence
C. SD → Consequence → Response
D. Consequence → Response → SD

15. Which is the **best** example of a clear SD for DTT?
A. "Do the thing we talked about"
B. "Can you show me something cool?"
C. "Touch the car"
D. "You know what to do, right?"

16. Which scenario best illustrates Natural Environment Teaching (NET)?
A. Drilling vocabulary words at a table with no toys
B. Practicing colors with flashcards only
C. Prompting the child to request "bubbles" during a bubble play activity they enjoy
D. Requiring the child to write words for 30 minutes silently

17. A BCBA sets up a backward chain for handwashing. Which step will the learner typically complete independently first?
A. The first step (turn on water)
B. The last step (dry hands/turn off water)
C. A random step in the middle
D. All steps at once

18. Shaping is best described as:
A. Teaching a long chain of behaviors step-by-step
B. Reinforcing successive approximations toward a final target behavior
C. Ignoring all behavior until the perfect response occurs
D. Giving reinforcement on a fixed schedule only

19. A plan says to start with a model prompt and then move to a gestural prompt, then to no prompt as the client improves. This is an example of:
A. Reinforcement thinning
B. Prompt fading
C. Extinction
D. DRO

20. Which statement about reinforcement is most accurate?
A. Any reward will work as reinforcement
B. Reinforcement is anything the RBT likes
C. Reinforcement increases the future likelihood of a behavior
D. Reinforcement means giving a child candy

21. A BCBA determines that a child's hitting is maintained by escape from tasks. Which replacement behavior is the most functionally equivalent?
A. Saying "hi" to peers
B. Clapping hands
C. Asking for a break appropriately

D. Laughing quietly

22. A plan to reduce behavior by removing the reinforcement that used to follow it is called:
    A. Extinction
    B. Shaping
    C. Chaining
    D. Prompting
23. When extinction is first implemented, which effect is most likely?
    A. Behavior immediately stops and disappears
    B. Behavior temporarily increases in intensity or frequency
    C. Behavior never changes at all
    D. Behavior turns into a different diagnosis
24. DRA (Differential Reinforcement of Alternative behavior) means:
    A. Reinforcing any behavior except the problem behavior
    B. Reinforcing a specific alternative behavior and not the problem behavior
    C. Reinforcing the problem behavior occasionally
    D. Punishing the problem behavior only
25. DRO (Differential Reinforcement of Other behavior) means:
    A. Reinforcing the problem behavior after it happens
    B. Reinforcing any behavior that is dangerous
    C. Providing reinforcement if the problem behavior does **not** occur during a set interval
    D. Ignoring all behavior for a day
26. Which of the following best describes the **RBT's role** in behavior reduction?
    A. Designing new reduction procedures independently
    B. Implementing the written plan and collecting accurate data
    C. Deciding which punishers to use
    D. Changing the plan when parents complain
27. A client engages in severe self-injury. The plan includes a specific protective hold that you have **not** been trained to use. What should you do?
    A. Attempt the hold anyway by copying the written description
    B. Ask another untrained staff to help you use it
    C. Inform your supervisor that you are not trained and use only procedures you are trained and authorized to use
    D. Invent your own restraint
28. Which note is the **most objective**?
    A. "The client was awful and rude today."
    B. "Client hates therapy and is manipulative."
    C. "Client kicked the table 4 times during math work and shouted 'no' twice."
    D. "The client clearly doesn't like me."
29. After a minor injury (small scratch) that occurred when a client fell, and safety has been handled, what is the **best** next step?
    A. Ignore it since it was minor
    B. Document the incident factually and follow your organization's reporting procedures
    C. Change the behavior plan yourself
    D. Tell only other RBTs informally

30. Which is an example of a **variable that may affect the client** and should be documented?
    A. The RBT forgot their lunch
    B. The client's parent reports the child did not sleep the night before
    C. The clinic is repainting next year
    D. The RBT plans a vacation in 6 months
31. Which action best protects client confidentiality?
    A. Discussing a client's behavior in a crowded elevator
    B. Leaving session notes on a shared break room table
    C. Keeping paper records in a locked cabinet when not in use
    D. Sharing session details with friends to get advice
32. A teacher asks, "What goals did you work on with this student today?" What is an appropriate RBT response?
    A. "I can't tell you anything."
    B. "We practiced following two-step directions; they completed 7 of 10 independently."
    C. "The student is terrible during sessions."
    D. "I'll change the goals to what you want tomorrow."
33. A parent asks you, "Do you think we should change my child's medication dose?" What is the **best** response?
    A. Give advice based on other clients' experiences
    B. Say it's not your role to give medical advice and suggest they talk with their doctor and BCBA
    C. Adjust the dose yourself
    D. Tell them it doesn't matter
34. A coworker says they never record minor problem behaviors because "it takes too long." What should you do?
    A. Also stop recording them to match
    B. Destroy your old data so they match
    C. Continue documenting as required and share the concern with your supervisor
    D. Yell at the coworker in front of clients
35. A parent asks you to "use spanking if he hits you," even though this is not in the plan and your agency forbids it. What should you do?
    A. Agree in secret
    B. Spank only lightly
    C. Explain that you must follow the written plan and cannot use physical punishment, then inform your supervisor
    D. Ask another staff member to do it
36. Which task is **within** the RBT's scope of practice?
    A. Conducting a full functional analysis alone
    B. Writing and approving behavior plans
    C. Implementing programs and collecting data as written by the supervisor
    D. Changing treatment goals based on personal judgment
37. A BCBA schedules supervision time to review your work. What is the most professional way to use that time?
    A. Show up without data or questions
    B. Arrive prepared with data, questions, and examples of challenges
    C. Refuse to attend because you feel confident
    D. Use the time to gossip about families

38. A teacher wants you to "ignore the BCBA's plan" and use a different strategy, but the BCBA has not approved a change. What should you do?
    A. Do what the teacher says to avoid conflict
    B. Mix both plans however you like
    C. Explain you must follow the BCBA's plan and offer to have the BCBA speak with the teacher
    D. Stop running any program at all
39. A parent invites you to be their child's regular babysitter on weekends. What is the most appropriate response?
    A. Accept for extra income
    B. Accept as long as you don't mention ABA
    C. Politely decline and explain that this creates a dual relationship and is not appropriate
    D. Agree, as long as the BCBA doesn't find out
40. Which example shows **professional, objective documentation** of a session?
    A. "Client was good; nothing to report."
    B. "Client completed 9 of 10 trials of the requesting program independently; one brief aggression incident (pushing peer) occurred during cleanup."
    C. "The client was super annoying today."
    D. "Client definitely hates therapy and doesn't try."
41. On a simple line graph of behavior, what is usually shown on the horizontal (x) axis?
    A. The type of reinforcer
    B. Time or sessions
    C. The client's age
    D. The number of staff
42. The vertical (y) axis on a behavior graph most often shows:
    A. The amount or level of the behavior (e.g., frequency, rate, percentage)
    B. Names of staff
    C. Dates of supervision meetings
    D. The client's diagnosis
43. A graph shows that the number of aggressive incidents per day has steadily decreased over the last two weeks. Which statement best describes this trend?
    A. Increasing trend
    B. Decreasing trend
    C. Flat trend
    D. High variability with no pattern
44. Two RBTs observe the same session using the same definition of "tantrum." Their data are very similar. This mainly shows:
    A. High treatment integrity
    B. Good interobserver agreement (reliability)
    C. Poor operational definitions
    D. That behavior is definitely improving
45. A client's behavior suddenly worsens and becomes more intense. The parent tells you the family recently moved and the child is not sleeping well. What should you do?
    A. Ignore this information
    B. Tell the parent the move was a bad choice

C. Document these variables and inform your supervisor
D. Change the plan yourself

46. During a session, a client engages in severe aggression requiring you to use crisis procedures. After safety is handled, what should you do next?
A. Hide the incident so no one is upset
B. Document the event objectively and contact your supervisor promptly
C. Stop all future sessions without telling anyone
D. Punish the client later

47. Why is it important to read exam questions carefully, especially words like "first," "best," or "most ethical"?
A. Because those words often change which answer is correct
B. So you can memorize the questions
C. So you can answer faster
D. So you can skip reading the options

48. During the RBT exam, if you don't know an answer and guessing is not penalized, what should you do?
A. Leave it blank
B. Randomly pick A for all such questions
C. Eliminate clearly wrong options and make your best guess
D. Spend 10 minutes on that one question

49. Which mindset is most helpful on RBT exam day?
A. "If I miss one question, I've already failed."
B. "I've prepared; I need to read carefully and choose the best answer for each question."
C. "It doesn't matter; I won't study."
D. "I should change every answer at least once."

50. Why should an RBT understand the overall RBT Task List and exam content areas?
A. So they can challenge the BACB
B. So they know exactly what is outside their role and what skills they are accountable for
C. So they can diagnose and treat independently
D. So they never need supervision

51. A BCBA asks you to start a new data sheet today. You don't fully understand how to fill it out. What is the **best** thing to do?
A. Guess how to use it and hope it's right
B. Ask your supervisor for clarification before using it
C. Ignore it and keep using the old one
D. Make your own version without telling anyone

52. A parent is upset and says, "Therapy is making my child worse. You need to stop the program today." What should you do?
A. Immediately stop all programs permanently
B. Argue with the parent and tell them they're wrong
C. Listen respectfully, explain that treatment decisions are made by the BCBA, and let the supervisor know right away
D. Ignore the parent and continue as usual

53. Which of the following situations is **most likely** to require an incident report?
A. The client refused a snack
B. The client changed preferred toy

C. The client scratched another child hard enough to cause bleeding

D. The client did not complete all tasks

54. A client appears suddenly very lethargic and different from usual. The parent reports a new medication started yesterday. What should you do?

A. Ignore it because medication is not your concern

B. Tell the parent to stop the medication

C. Document what you observe and what the parent reported, and inform your supervisor

D. Diagnose a side effect

55. Your supervisor asks you to collect data on self-injury using frequency and duration. What is your responsibility?

A. Decide to use a different method if it seems easier

B. Collect frequency and duration as instructed and ask questions if you are unsure

C. Only collect data when behavior looks severe

D. Let another staff guess the numbers

56. Which is the **best** example of maintaining client dignity?

A. Laughing when a client has a meltdown because it looks funny

B. Talking about the client's behavior loudly in a public hallway

C. Offering choices when possible and speaking respectfully even when behavior is challenging

D. Ignoring the client when they speak

57. A family's cultural practices include specific greetings and ways of addressing adults. As an RBT, what should you do?

A. Insist that your way is the only correct way

B. Refuse to participate in greetings

C. Respect their customs as long as they don't conflict with safety or ethics, and discuss any questions with your supervisor

D. Tell the family to change their culture

58. A client is crying and pushing materials away during a non-essential task, and appears clearly distressed. The plan allows for choice and breaks. What is the most appropriate action?

A. Force the client to finish the task no matter what

B. Offer a break or alternative activity as allowed in the plan

C. Yell at the client to stop crying

D. Ignore the distress until the end of the session

59. Which of the following best shows assent (willing participation) from a client?

A. The client calmly joins the activity and follows along without resistance

B. The client screams and tries to leave

C. The client hides under the table when you arrive

D. The client repeatedly says "no" to every instruction

60. A parent asks you to send session videos to their personal social media so relatives can watch. Your agency prohibits this. What should you do?

A. Agree and send videos anyway

B. Edit the videos and then send

C. Explain that sharing videos that way is against policy and suggest they talk to the supervisor about approved options

D. Upload them anonymously

61. Which of the following is an example of **treatment integrity** (fidelity)?
    A. The RBT skips steps when busy
    B. The RBT implements all steps of the behavior plan as written during the session
    C. The parent changes the plan daily
    D. The RBT guesses which prompts to use
62. An RBT consistently arrives 15–20 minutes late to sessions without notice. Which concern does this most directly raise?
    A. Data collection methods
    B. Professionalism and reliability
    C. Graphing skills
    D. Preference assessment
63. A BCBA asks you to practice a new prompting procedure with them before using it with the client. Why is this important?
    A. It wastes time
    B. It allows you to demonstrate and receive feedback so you implement it correctly
    C. It lets you change the plan
    D. It replaces data collection
64. Which of the following is **outside** the RBT's role?
    A. Taking ABC data
    B. Running a preference assessment
    C. Designing a new functional analysis from scratch
    D. Collecting frequency data on target behavior
65. A client makes a rude comment about your appearance. What is the most professional response?
    A. Argue with the client
    B. Make fun of the client in return
    C. Remain calm, follow the plan for responding to such behavior, and continue the session professionally
    D. Quit on the spot
66. A coworker posts a photo on social media that clearly shows a client's face during a session. What is your best action?
    A. Like and share the post
    B. Ignore it because it's not your account
    C. Report the concern to your supervisor or appropriate compliance contact
    D. Comment with the client's full name
67. Which of the following best describes **scope of competence** for an RBT?
    A. The RBT can do anything as long as they feel confident
    B. The RBT should only perform tasks they have been trained and are competent to do under supervision
    C. The RBT can diagnose clients in emergencies
    D. The RBT can modify plans without training
68. A caregiver requests to "skip data today because we are in a hurry." What should you do?
    A. Agree and skip data collection
    B. Tell them that data collection is required as part of services and continue as planned, or consult your supervisor if needed
    C. Fake the data later
    D. Let the caregiver fill in random numbers

69. Which statement about **interobserver agreement (IOA)** is true?
    A. It measures how long behavior lasts
    B. It shows how consistent data are between two or more observers
    C. It is only needed for graphs
    D. It is a type of punishment
70. A client is receiving services at school and at home. Why is consistent communication between teams important?
    A. So staff can complain about families
    B. To coordinate strategies and share relevant progress while staying in each person's role
    C. To make teachers follow ABA at all times
    D. To avoid collecting data
71. A BCBA from another agency calls and asks for detailed information about your client. There is no signed release of information on file. What should you do?
    A. Share everything to help the child
    B. Share only the diagnosis
    C. Explain you cannot share information without proper authorization and refer them to your supervisor
    D. Email them your notes from your personal account
72. During a session, you realize you forgot to bring a required visual schedule. What is the **best** response?
    A. Make up a completely different system without telling anyone
    B. Do your best to approximate the procedure using available materials, document the change, and notify your supervisor
    C. Cancel the session immediately
    D. Pretend the schedule is not important
73. A client has mastered a skill, but you notice they are not using it at home. What should you do?
    A. Assume the parents are not trying
    B. Document what you observe/are told and discuss with your supervisor to plan for better generalization
    C. Remove the skill from the program
    D. Blame the client in your notes
74. Which is an appropriate way to support **generalization** of a new communication skill?
    A. Only practice the skill with one RBT in one room
    B. Practice the skill with different people, in different settings, and with different materials
    C. Stop practicing once the client does it once
    D. Practice only with unusual items
75. A parent says they don't want you to work on certain self-care skills due to their cultural values. What is the best response?
    A. Argue with them until they agree
    B. Ignore their concern and continue
    C. Respectfully listen, document the discussion, and refer the issue to your supervisor for further planning
    D. Remove all other goals
76. A client repeatedly asks for your personal phone number. What should you do?
    A. Give it to build rapport
    B. Ignore them and walk away
    C. Politely decline, explain that it's not appropriate, and redirect to a program or appropriate topic
    D. Tell them to ask another staff

77. Why is accurate **time-in/time-out** recording (session start and end times) important?
    A. It is only for your paycheck
    B. It affects billing, documentation, and accurate interpretation of rate-based data
    C. It replaces behavior data
    D. It is optional
78. When graphing rate, which combination is most accurate?
    A. Total behaviors per day, ignoring time
    B. Behaviors per unit of time (e.g., per hour) on the y-axis and sessions/days on the x-axis
    C. The client's age on the y-axis and weight on the x-axis
    D. Only percentages on both axes
79. A BCBA shows you that your implementation of a procedure is different from what's written in the plan. What should you do?
    A. Insist that your way is better
    B. Listen, ask questions, and adjust your implementation to match the plan
    C. Tell families the BCBA is wrong
    D. Refuse to change
80. Which of the following is the **best** RBT response when feeling overwhelmed by several challenging clients?
    A. Start cancelling sessions without notice
    B. Vent about clients on social media
    C. Talk with your supervisor about your workload and ask for guidance or support
    D. Stop collecting data
81. A school staff member asks you to share the full details of another client's behavior plan "for ideas." What should you do?
    A. Share the full plan
    B. Share a summary with names removed
    C. Explain that you can't share other clients' private plans and suggest they consult their own support team
    D. Email the plan to their personal account
82. Which scenario best reflects **professional boundaries** with coworkers?
    A. Frequently discussing client details in a public café
    B. Becoming close friends and sharing client gossip
    C. Maintaining friendly, respectful interactions while keeping client information private and work-focused
    D. Refusing to speak to coworkers at all
83. During an observation, your BCBA notes that you are very late delivering reinforcement after correct responses. Why is this a problem?
    A. It makes data look better
    B. The client may associate reinforcement with other behaviors occurring during the delay
    C. It increases generalization
    D. It has no impact
84. A client's parent requests that you speak in their home language when possible and offers to teach you key phrases. This is consistent with your agency's policies. What is the best response?
    A. Refuse and say you only speak one language
    B. Agree to learn and use appropriate phrases as you are able, and inform your supervisor about the request
    C. Ask the parent to translate sessions themselves
    D. Stop seeing the client

85. Why is it important for RBTs to seek clarification when they are unsure about a procedure?
    A. So they can avoid doing any work
    B. So they do not waste time reading plans
    C. So they can implement procedures accurately, maintain treatment integrity, and protect client welfare
    D. So they can take over the supervisor's role

Answer Key – Mock Exam A (with Brief Justifications)

1. B – Specific, observable definition = operational definition.
2. B – Counting each elopement over time = frequency/rate.
3. B – Duration = how long the work period lasts.
4. B – Latency = time from SD to response.
5. B – "Yes" if behavior occurs at any time in interval = partial-interval.
6. D – Check at the end of the interval = momentary time sampling.
7. C – Completed chores are a permanent product.
8. B – Free-operant preference = free access while you observe.
9. B – Paired-choice = two items at a time, record choice.
10. A – "A" = Antecedent.
11. C – "No more juice" happens right before behavior = antecedent.
12. C – Observing and recording during a session is direct assessment.
13. B – Baseline probe checks skill level before teaching.
14. B – DTT trial: SD → Response → Consequence.
15. C – "Touch the car" is clear and specific.
16. C – NET uses natural, motivating activities to teach.
17. B – Backward chaining teaches the last step first.
18. B – Shaping = reinforcing successive approximations.
19. B – Prompt fading gradually reduces prompts.
20. C – Reinforcement increases future likelihood of behavior.
21. C – Asking for a break also results in escape.
22. A – Extinction = remove maintaining reinforcement.
23. B – Extinction often causes a temporary increase (burst).
24. B – DRA reinforces a specific alternative behavior.
25. C – DRO reinforces the absence of the problem behavior in an interval.
26. B – RBT implements and records; doesn't design reduction plans.
27. C – Only use procedures you're trained in; contact supervisor.
28. C – Concrete, countable description = objective.
29. B – Document factually and follow incident procedures.
30. B – Lack of sleep can affect behavior; document it.
31. C – Locked cabinet protects confidentiality.
32. B – Neutral, session-based progress is appropriate.
33. B – Medical advice is outside scope; refer to doctor/BCBA.
34. C – Keep following requirements; report issue to supervisor.
35. C – Must follow plan and policy; no physical punishment.
36. C – Implementing programs and collecting data is in scope.
37. B – Coming prepared and engaged is professional.
38. C – Follow BCBA's plan and route concerns to them.
39. C – Babysitting is a dual relationship; politely decline.
40. B – Specific skill and behavior info = good documentation.
41. B – X-axis usually shows time or sessions.

42. A – Y-axis shows level of behavior (rate, frequency, %).
43. B – Fewer incidents over time = decreasing trend.
44. B – Similar data between observers = good IOA (reliability).
45. C – Document variables (move, sleep) and inform supervisor.
46. B – After safety: document objectively and contact supervisor.
47. A – Words like "first" and "best" change the correct answer.
48. C – Remove clearly wrong options and guess.
49. B – Calm, realistic approach focusing on careful reading helps.
50. B – Knowing the Task List clarifies responsibilities and limits.
51. B – Ask for clarification to use the data sheet correctly.
52. C – Respectful listening + involve BCBA for treatment decisions.
53. C – Injury to another child typically requires an incident report.
54. C – Document and inform supervisor; no medical advice.
55. B – Use the requested methods; ask if unsure.
56. C – Respectful language and offering choices supports dignity.
57. C – Respect cultural practices consistent with ethics; consult supervisor.
58. B – Use breaks/choices as allowed to reduce distress.
59. A – Calm, willing participation = assent.
60. C – Must follow policy and refer family to supervisor for options.
61. B – Treatment integrity = following plan as written.
62. B – Chronic lateness is a professionalism issue.
63. B – Practice and feedback ensure correct implementation.
64. C – Designing functional analysis is outside the RBT role.
65. C – Stay calm and follow the plan; remain professional.
66. C – Report confidentiality breach to supervisor/compliance contact.
67. B – RBTs should stay within trained, supervised tasks.
68. B – Data is required; explain and/or consult the supervisor.
69. B – IOA measures agreement between observers' data.
70. B – Communication helps coordinate strategies appropriately.
71. C – No release = no sharing; refer to supervisor.
72. B – Approximate, document deviation, and notify supervisor.
73. B – Document and discuss generalization issues with BCBA.
74. B – Varying people, settings, items promotes generalization.
75. C – Respectfully listen, document, and involve your supervisor.
76. C – Decline, explain boundary, and redirect.
77. B – Accurate time records affect billing and rate calculations.
78. B – Rate = behavior per time on y-axis, time/sessions on x-axis.
79. B – Adjust practice to match the written plan.
80. C – Talk with the supervisor when overwhelmed.
81. C – You can't share other clients' plans; protect privacy.
82. C – Friendly, respectful, and private about client info.
83. B – Delayed reinforcement may strengthen other behaviors.
84. B – Learning and using key phrases is respectful; inform the supervisor.
85. C – Clarification supports accurate implementation and client safety.

Mock RBT Practice Exam B (85 Questions)

Instructions

- This is a second full-length mock exam to give you **more practice** with RBT-style questions.
  - There are **85 multiple-choice questions**. Each has **one best answer**.
- Choose the **single best answer (A, B, C, or D)** for each item.
- Read carefully for key words like "first," "best," or "most appropriate," which often decide the correct answer.
- Use this exam to:
  - Practice timing and pacing, and/or
  - Diagnose weak areas to revisit in the chapters
- After you finish, use the **answer key** to check your work and review the justifications.

Questions

1. A supervisor defines "property destruction" as "throwing, kicking, or breaking objects with enough force that they move more than 6 inches or are damaged." This definition is:
   A. Too vague to measure
   B. An operational definition
   C. A diagnosis
   D. A reinforcement plan
2. For a behavior that has a clear beginning and end and occurs only a few times per day, the **simplest** appropriate measurement is:
   A. Frequency
   B. Duration
   C. Latency
   D. Whole-interval recording
3. A BCBA wants to measure how long each instance of "on-task behavior" lasts once it starts. Which measurement is best?
   A. Frequency
   B. Duration
   C. Latency
   D. Momentary time sampling
4. A plan says, "Record how long it takes from 'Line up please' until the client stands in line." What are you measuring?
   A. Rate
   B. Duration
   C. Latency
   D. Percentage
5. A behavior occurs so constantly that you cannot tell when one instance stops and another starts. Your supervisor divides the session into 30-second intervals and wants to know if the behavior happens at **any** time

in each interval. Which method is this?
A. Whole-interval recording
B. Partial-interval recording
C. Momentary time sampling
D. Time-delay prompting

6. In whole-interval recording, an interval is counted as "yes" if:
A. The behavior occurs at least once during the interval
B. The behavior occurs exactly at the end of the interval
C. The behavior occurs for the entire duration of the interval
D. The behavior occurs exactly 5 times

7. A teacher wants to know what percentage of time a student is on-task during a 20-minute activity. Which method would most directly give this information?
A. Duration of on-task behavior
B. Frequency of on-task responses
C. Whole-interval recording across the activity
D. Permanent product

8. Which example is **most clearly** permanent product measurement?
A. Counting how many minutes a client screams
B. Counting completed puzzle boards at the end of a session
C. Recording how often the client looks out the window
D. Observing whether the client is in their seat at the end of each minute

9. A free-operant preference assessment is characterized by:
A. Presenting one item at a time
B. Presenting two items at a time
C. Allowing free access to many items and observing engagement
D. Asking only the parent which item to use

10. In a single-stimulus (single-choice) preference assessment, the RBT:
A. Presents all items at once
B. Presents one item at a time and records approach or rejection
C. Avoids interacting with the client
D. Asks the client to rank items on a written list

11. A BCBA is exploring possible functions of aggression. They ask you to record what happens before and after each instance in natural settings. This is:
A. ABC descriptive assessment
B. Functional analysis
C. Baseline probing
D. Paired-choice assessment

12. In ABC data, which part is the **behavior**?
A. "Teacher says, 'Clean up time.'"
B. "Client throws blocks and yells, 'No!'"
C. "Teacher gives client a break."
D. "Teacher talks to parent after session."

13. Which of the following is an example of **indirect** assessment?
A. Frequency recording during session

B. ABC data collection
C. Parent interview about behavior
D. Momentary time sampling

14. Before teaching "brushing teeth," your supervisor wants to know which steps the client can already do independently. You follow a checklist of steps and record independent vs prompted performance. This is:
A. A task analysis
B. A skill assessment using a task analysis
C. A functional analysis
D. An extinction procedure

15. During DTT, the instruction "Give me red" is the:
A. Consequence
B. Prompt
C. SD
D. Replacement behavior

16. Which of the following is **most** like discrete-trial teaching?
A. Child roams freely and you occasionally comment on behavior
B. Short, repeated learning trials with clear SDs, defined responses, and programmed consequences
C. Only playing with no structure
D. Giving praise at random times

17. In Natural Environment Teaching (NET), teaching opportunities are:
A. Scripted and delivered at a table only
B. Embedded into play, routines, and activities the learner enjoys
C. Provided only after long lectures
D. Rarely connected to the child's interests

18. A forward chain for toothbrushing has been set up. Which step does the learner typically do independently first?
A. The first step in the chain
B. The last step in the chain
C. A random middle step
D. All steps at once

19. A BCBA wants to strengthen a new vocal response. At first, the client gets reinforcement for any vocalization, then only for approximations like "much," and finally only for saying "more." This is:
A. Chaining
B. Shaping
C. Extinction
D. DRO

20. Which is the **best** description of a prompt?
A. Any reward given after correct behavior
B. A temporary extra cue that helps the learner produce the correct response
C. A type of punishment
D. A type of reinforcer

21. An example of a **response prompt** is:
A. Moving a worksheet closer to the learner
B. Saying, "Touch the dog" while pointing to the dog

C. Changing the lighting in the room
D. Rearranging chairs

22. An example of a **stimulus prompt** is:
A. Physically guiding the learner's hand
B. Saying the correct answer quietly
C. Highlighting the correct picture with a colored border
D. Modeling the response yourself
23. A plan states that the RBT will gradually remove physical guidance and move to a light touch, then no touch, while the client keeps responding correctly. This is:
A. Prompt fading
B. Reinforcer thinning
C. Extinction
D. DRO
24. A parent offers the child a preferred game after finishing homework. The next day, the child finishes homework more quickly. The game functioned as:
A. Punishment
B. Extinction
C. Reinforcement
D. Baseline
25. A client screams until they are given a tablet. Screaming then happens more often in the future. The most likely function is:
A. Automatic (sensory)
B. Attention
C. Tangibles (access to items)
D. Escape
26. A client bangs their head when given hard math problems, and the tasks are usually removed. The most likely function is:
A. Escape
B. Attention
C. Tangibles
D. Automatic
27. A plan to reduce behavior includes: teaching a break card, reinforcing its use, and continuing the task when problem behavior occurs. This plan is using:
A. Reinforcement only
B. Extinction only
C. Replacement behavior plus extinction for problem behavior
D. Punishment only
28. DRI (Differential Reinforcement of Incompatible behavior) means reinforcing a behavior that:
A. Is less frequent than the problem behavior
B. Cannot occur at the same time as the problem behavior
C. Happens after the problem behavior
D. Is always off-task
29. Which of the following is **most likely** an incompatible behavior for "running out of the room"?
A. Shouting

B. Sitting in a chair with feet on the floor
C. Asking for help
D. Complaining quietly

30. A plan says, "If no aggression occurs for 5 minutes, deliver praise and a token." This is:
A. DRA
B. DRO
C. DRI
D. Extinction

31. A consequence that **decreases** the future likelihood of a behavior is called:
A. Reinforcement
B. Punishment
C. Extinction
D. Shaping

32. Which is an example of negative reinforcement?
A. Child earns a sticker for raising hand
B. Child is given extra chores after yelling
C. Task is removed after a child appropriately asks for a break, and asking for breaks increases
D. Child loses points after being rude

33. A BCBA adds a time-out procedure to a plan. As an RBT, your responsibility is to:
A. Decide when to use time-out based on your feelings
B. Implement time-out exactly as written and trained, and collect data
C. Rewrite the time-out rules
D. Avoid using it because you disagree

34. Which note is **most** objective and appropriate?
A. "Client is a brat when others are present."
B. "Client was angry all session."
C. "The client shouted 'no' three times and threw a pencil once during a writing task."
D. "Client hates handwriting."

35. After a serious incident where a client hit another student, what should you do once safety is restored?
A. Say nothing, so no one gets in trouble
B. Document the incident objectively and follow incident reporting procedures
C. Delete the data for the day
D. Blame the other student in your notes

36. Which is an example of a **relevant** variable that may affect the client?
A. The RBT's favorite TV show was canceled
B. The client's sibling moved out of the home last week
C. The RBT is hungry
D. A new coffee machine arrived at the clinic

37. Which statement best describes **objective documentation**?
A. It describes what happened in measurable, observable terms
B. It includes the RBT's personal feelings
C. It focuses on who is to blame
D. It uses emotional language

38. Which action helps protect confidentiality?

A. Talking about clients at a restaurant with coworkers
B. Taking pictures of session notes on your personal phone
C. Keeping electronic records in password-protected systems
D. Leaving files open on a shared computer

39. A teacher asks, "Can you tell me generally how the student did today?" What is the **best** response?
A. "They were awful."
B. "They completed 80% of their independent work with minimal prompts and had one brief episode of yelling during transitions."
C. "I'm not allowed to say anything to you."
D. "The BCBA is doing everything wrong."

40. A parent asks what they can do at home to support a new communication skill you're teaching. As an RBT you should:
A. Say, "I can't talk to you about that."
B. Give them detailed ABA theory
C. Share simple strategies from the plan that you are trained to explain and suggest they discuss further with the BCBA
D. Tell them to do whatever they want

41. A parent says, "I'm thinking of stopping services next week." What should you do?
A. Promise them that behavior will improve immediately
B. Argue with them
C. Listen respectfully, document the concern, and inform your supervisor promptly
D. Ignore the comment

42. Which of the following actions violates RBT boundaries?
A. Saying hello to a client in public if they approach
B. Accepting expensive gifts from a client's family
C. Explaining session activities in neutral terms
D. Attending scheduled meetings with the BCBA

43. A parent offers you concert tickets worth several hundred dollars. Your organization prohibits valuable gifts. What is the **best** response?
A. Accept but don't tell anyone
B. Accept and give the tickets to another RBT
C. Politely decline, explain the policy, and inform your supervisor
D. Sell the tickets and buy toys

44. An RBT discusses a client's detailed behavior history in a crowded waiting room where others can overhear. This is primarily a problem with:
A. Data collection
B. Confidentiality and professionalism
C. Graphing skills
D. Reinforcement delivery

45. Which task is a **core** RBT responsibility?
A. Writing treatment goals
B. Conducting diagnostic evaluations
C. Implementing skill-acquisition and behavior-reduction plans under supervision
D. Approving plans for insurance

46. A BCBA asks you to take frequency data on a new behavior starting today. What should you do?
    A. Decide to use duration data instead
    B. Collect frequency data as requested and clarify any questions
    C. Ignore the request
    D. Ask another RBT to make up numbers
47. During supervision, your BCBA gives you feedback that you are rushing through trials and not giving the client enough time to respond. What is the most appropriate reaction?
    A. Argue and say they are wrong
    B. Listen, ask for examples, and practice giving sufficient wait time
    C. Quit the job
    D. Ignore the feedback
48. A coworker consistently fails to follow the behavior plan and uses threats instead. What should you do?
    A. Join them so the client hears a consistent message
    B. Secretly change the plan
    C. Continue to follow the plan yourself and report your concerns to your supervisor
    D. Yell at the coworker in front of clients
49. A client is receiving speech therapy and ABA services. What should you think about the speech therapist's role?
    A. As a competitor
    B. As another professional with expertise who can collaborate with your BCBA
    C. As someone you should ignore
    D. As your assistant
50. A teacher asks you to recommend a diagnosis for a student. What should you say?
    A. Provide a diagnosis based on your experience
    B. Tell them that diagnoses are outside your role and refer them to appropriate professionals
    C. Make a guess and write it down
    D. Ask the parent to choose a diagnosis
51. Which is the **best** example of professional language about a client?
    A. "They are super lazy."
    B. "They completed 5 out of 7 tasks with verbal prompts."
    C. "They are impossible."
    D. "They just don't care."
52. A client's parent asks you to attend a family party as a guest. This would most likely:
    A. Create a dual relationship
    B. Be required
    C. Be part of treatment integrity
    D. Improve IOA
53. An RBT notices that a client's behavior is very different when a particular staff member is present. What is the **best** thing to do?
    A. Accuse the staff member directly in front of others
    B. Ignore it
    C. Document observations and share them with the supervisor during supervision
    D. Change the schedule yourself
54. A BCBA asks you to help with a structured skills assessment. Your role is likely to be:

A. Choosing which assessment tool to use
B. Interpreting the assessment results
C. Administering tasks and recording responses as trained
D. Diagnosing the client

55. Which of the following is an appropriate **hand-off** to the next RBT at the end of your session?
A. "Good luck, they were awful."
B. "Client had one tantrum during transitions; we followed the plan, and data are on the sheet. They did well on requesting the program—8/10 independent."
C. "You'll see, I'm not telling you anything."
D. "Just do whatever you want."

56. A BCBA is required to observe your work regularly. This is mainly because:
A. They don't trust RBTs
B. They must supervise, monitor treatment integrity, and provide feedback
C. They are trying to get you in trouble
D. It is only for billing

57. Which is an example of **generalization** of a skill?
A. Client uses a new request only with one RBT in one room
B. Client uses a new request with parents, teachers, and RBTs in several settings
C. Client stops using the skill
D. Client only uses the skill when bribed

58. A client who has learned to mand (request) for items now begins to use that skill in a different classroom without prompting. This is an example of:
A. Maintenance
B. Generalization
C. Extinction
D. Shaping

59. A BCBA asks you to help measure whether a skill is maintained after teaching ends. Which is most appropriate?
A. Stop testing the skill entirely
B. Occasionally probe the skill after it is "mastered" to see if it still occurs
C. Delete all data
D. Only measure problem behaviors

60. A client meets mastery criteria on a program. What is the RBT's role?
A. Decide independently to remove the program
B. Continue implementing or probing the program according to the BCBA's instructions
C. Write new goals
D. Change reinforcement schedules alone

61. An RBT is feeling sick but shows up to work with a contagious illness. This primarily violates:
A. Graphing guidelines
B. Professional conduct and client welfare
C. Reinforcer selection
D. IOA procedures

62. Why is it important to maintain accurate, honest data even when behavior looks "bad"?
A. To avoid getting caught

B. So the BCBA can make real, data-based decisions and not rely on false information
C. So the client looks worse
D. So you can prove you are right

63. A coworker suggests "just rounding up the data to make the graph look better." What should you do?
A. Agree to keep it simple
B. Continue recording accurately, refuse to falsify data, and report the concern to your supervisor
C. Let them do it for you
D. Round even more

64. A client becomes upset when they see new staff. The BCBA asks you to take latency data on "time from new staff entering the room to the first instance of crying." Your primary job is to:
A. Decide the function of crying
B. Diagnose anxiety
C. Use a timer to measure latency as instructed and record accurately
D. Change the environment yourself

65. Which is an example of a **permanent product** related to self-help skills?
A. Duration of toothbrushing
B. Number of clothing items correctly folded and put away
C. Frequency of prompts to brush teeth
D. Percentage of on-task behavior

66. A teacher asks you to sign a document stating the student no longer needs any accommodations. You are unsure. What should you do?
A. Sign it to be polite
B. Refuse and argue
C. Explain you cannot sign such documents and refer them to your supervisor or appropriate school staff
D. Ask the student to sign instead

67. A client's parent requests daily communication. What can you appropriately share as an RBT?
A. Detailed opinions about the client's personality
B. Objective summaries of session activities and progress, consistent with the plan and agency policy
C. Other clients' information for comparison
D. Your personal life details

68. Which is the **best** example of an objective session summary?
A. "The client was super difficult and annoying."
B. "Client clearly hates the program."
C. "Client completed 12 of 15 trials independently on the manding program; one tantrum occurred when denied tablet access."
D. "Client is probably regressing."

69. A new RBT joins the team and asks you to share your login credentials so they can access the data system. What should you do?
A. Share as long as you trust them
B. Write it on the whiteboard
C. Refuse to share and tell them to obtain their own login through proper channels
D. Give them partial access

70. Why should RBTs avoid dual relationships with clients and families?
A. It makes work less fun

B. It can impair professional judgment and blur boundaries
C. It improves data
D. It makes billing easier

71. A BCBA asks if you are comfortable with a new physical prompting procedure and offers additional training. You are not fully comfortable yet. What is the **best** response?
A. Pretend you are comfortable and start anyway
B. Admit you need more training before using it with clients
C. Refuse all training
D. Ask another RBT to do it without training

72. During a home session, a caregiver starts yelling at the child in a way that seems abusive. What should you do **first**?
A. Join in to increase control
B. Immediately confront the caregiver aggressively
C. Prioritize the client's immediate safety and follow your organization's policies (which may include removing the client from harm and contacting your supervisor or mandated reporting line)
D. Ignore it

73. Which of the following is **most likely** to be included in an RBT's documentation if they suspect abuse?
A. Personal opinions and guesses
B. Emotional comments about the caregiver
C. Objective notes about what was directly observed or disclosed, following policy
D. Diagnoses about the caregiver

74. An RBT is unsure whether a situation is reportable as abuse. What is the best step?
A. Do nothing
B. Post about it online to get opinions
C. Consult with their supervisor or follow agency policies for mandated reporters
D. Ask the client to decide

75. A BCBA wants to see if a new schedule changes behavior. They ask you to continue the same measurement as before and not change methods mid-study. Why?
A. To keep it boring
B. So data are comparable across time
C. To confuse insurance
D. To make you do more work

76. Which kind of question is the RBT exam MOST likely to ask?
A. Essay questions about theory
B. Multiple-choice questions with applied scenarios
C. Long calculations with formulas
D. Open-ended treatment planning

77. Why is it important to pace yourself during the exam?
A. So you can finish as fast as possible with no thought
B. To avoid running out of time before answering all questions
C. Because pacing affects your score directly
D. Because the BACB requires walking breaks

78. If you encounter a very difficult question on the exam, a good strategy is to:
A. Spend most of your time on it

B. Panic and leave the test
C. Make your best choice, mark it (if allowed), move on, and return if time remains
D. Skip all remaining questions

79. When two answers seem good, the one that is usually correct on the RBT exam is the one that:
A. Gives the RBT more power
B. Follows the written plan, respects scope, protects client rights, and uses supervision
C. Saves staff time
D. Is most convenient for caregivers, regardless of the plan

80. After failing a practice exam, the best response is to:
A. Give up on the real exam
B. Use the results to identify weak areas and focus your studying
C. Ignore the score
D. Take the real exam immediately without review

81. Why is it risky to rely only on "common sense" for ethics questions?
A. The exam doesn't have ethics questions
B. "Common sense" may not match specific ethical codes and scope requirements
C. Ethics are not important
D. RBTs can make up their own rules

82. A good way to prepare for scenario questions is to:
A. Only memorize definitions
B. Practice reading scenarios and explaining why each answer is right or wrong
C. Avoid practice questions
D. Focus only on graphs

83. The **primary** purpose of the RBT exam is to:
A. Test advanced BCBA-level theory
B. Ensure RBTs can safely and correctly perform their role under supervision
C. Eliminate most candidates
D. Choose supervisors

84. After passing the RBT exam, your learning:
A. Is complete; you no longer need feedback
B. Continues through supervision and experience with clients
C. Replaces the need for supervision
D. Allows you to diagnose and treat independently

85. Overall, which combination best supports success as an RBT and on the exam?
A. Luck, guessing, and no studying
B. Content knowledge, realistic practice with scenarios, and following ethics and supervision structures
C. Ignoring data and going with your feelings
D. Changing plans without telling anyone

Answer Key – Mock Exam B (with Brief Justifications)

1. B – Specific, observable, measurable description = operational definition.
2. A – For a low-frequency, clear behavior, frequency is the simplest choice.
3. B – Duration measures how long on-task behavior lasts.
4. C – Latency = time from instruction to start of response.
5. B – "Any time in the interval" = partial-interval recording.
6. C – Whole-interval counts "yes" only if behavior occurs the entire interval.
7. C – Whole-interval across activity helps estimate percent time on-task.
8. B – Completed puzzles are a permanent product.
9. C – Free-operant preference allows free access while you observe engagement.
10. B – Single-stimulus: one item at a time, record approach/reject.
11. A – Recording antecedent and consequence = ABC descriptive assessment.
12. B – Behavior is the actual response (throwing blocks and yelling).
13. C – Parent interview is indirect assessment.
14. B – You're using a task analysis as a skill assessment checklist.
15. C – The instruction "Give me red" is the SD.
16. B – DTT uses short, structured trials with clear SDs and consequences.
17. B – NET embeds teaching in natural activities and play.
18. A – Forward chaining teaches the first step independently first.
19. B – Reinforcing closer approximations from "any sound" to "more" = shaping.
20. B – A prompt is a temporary extra cue to help evoke the correct response.
21. B – Pointing along with saying the SD is a response prompt (extra cue on the response).
22. C – Highlighting the correct picture is a stimulus prompt (altering the stimulus).
23. A – Gradual reduction in prompt intrusiveness is prompt fading.
24. C – The game increased homework behavior = reinforcement.
25. C – Screaming gains tablet access; function is tangible.
26. A – Task removal suggests escape-maintained behavior.
27. C – Teaching break cards + not letting problem behavior escape is replacement + extinction.
28. B – Incompatible behaviors cannot occur at the same time as problem behavior.
29. B – Sitting in a chair cannot happen while running out of the room.
30. B – Reinforcement after set time with no aggression = DRO.
31. B – Punishment reduces future likelihood of behavior.
32. C – Removal of a task after a proper break request, with breaks increasing, is negative reinforcement.
33. B – RBT must implement time-out as written and collect data, not alter it.
34. C – Describes specific actions and counts (objective).
35. B – Serious incidents need objective documentation and incident reporting.
36. B – A major family change can affect behavior and is relevant.
37. A – Objective documentation uses observable, measurable descriptions.
38. C – Password-protected records support confidentiality.
39. B – Neutral performance summary with data is appropriate.
40. C – RBT can share simple, plan-consistent strategies and refer to BCBA.
41. C – Listen, document, and inform BCBA promptly.

42. B – Accepting expensive gifts creates a boundary violation.
43. C – Decline, cite policy, and inform supervisor.
44. B – Discussing details in public violates confidentiality and professionalism.
45. C – RBTs implement plans and collect data under supervision.
46. B – Follow instructions, use frequency, clarify questions as needed.
47. B – Listen, ask for examples, and practice slowing down trials.
48. C – Continue following plan and report concerns to supervisor.
49. B – ST is a related profession; collaborate via BCBA.
50. B – Diagnoses are outside RBT scope; refer to appropriate professionals.
51. B – Concrete performance description is professional and objective.
52. A – Social invitations like family parties can create dual relationships.
53. C – Document and share observations with supervisor, not confront publicly.
54. C – RBT helps administer and record assessment tasks as trained.
55. B – Clear, descriptive hand-off with data and key events is appropriate.
56. B – BCBA must supervise, monitor fidelity, and provide feedback.
57. B – Using skill across people/settings = generalization.
58. B – Using the skill in a new classroom without prompts = generalization.
59. B – Occasional probes after mastery measure maintenance.
60. B – Continue or probe per BCBA's instructions, not remove independently.
61. B – Coming to work sick with something contagious risks client welfare.
62. B – Honest data allows real data-based decisions.
63. B – Refuse to falsify data and report concern; keep data accurate.
64. C – Your job is to measure latency accurately with a timer.
65. B – Folded clothes are a permanent product of self-help behavior.
66. C – RBT can't sign such documents; refer to supervisor/school team.
67. B – Objective, policy-consistent daily summaries are appropriate.
68. C – Specific performance + brief incident description is objective.
69. C – Never share login; tell them to get their own through proper channels.
70. B – Dual relationships can blur boundaries and impair judgment.
71. B – Being honest about needing more training protects clients and integrity.
72. C – Client safety comes first; follow policy and contact supervisor/mandated line.
73. C – Objective notes about what you saw/heard are required; avoid opinions.
74. C – When unsure, follow policy and consult supervisor/mandated reporting guidelines.
75. B – Same measurement method keeps data comparable.
76. B – RBT exam uses multiple-choice scenario questions.
77. B – Pacing helps ensure you answer all questions before time runs out.
78. C – Best strategy: make a choice, mark it, move on, return if possible.
79. B – The exam favors answers that follow the plan, ethics, and supervision.
80. B – Use practice results to focus study on weaker domains.
81. B – Ethics are code-based; "common sense" can conflict with actual rules.
82. B – Explaining why each option is right/wrong builds scenario skills.
83. B – Exam ensures you can safely perform the RBT role under supervision.
84. B – Certification is the beginning; learning continues with supervision and practice.
85. B – Knowledge + realistic practice + ethics/supervision = best success combo.

About the Author

CertiPrep Publishing specializes in high-quality certification exam prep books. We empower learners with expert resources to succeed in their professional certifications.

www.ingramcontent.com/pod-product-compliance
Lightning Source LLC
LaVergne TN
LVHW082353200926
848481LV00012B/3553